Drops of Reality 3

*New tales from a doctor's surgery
– and life experiences*

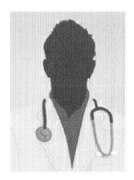

By Dr M. A. Moss

Drops of Reality 3
Independently published, 2020.
Copyright © Dr M. A. Moss, 2020.
ISBN: 9798673289846.

Book design and formatting: Jim Bruce, www.ebooklover.co.uk

Contents

Introduction

First I would like to thank my wonderful readers for their continued encouragement and positive feedback for the first two books in this series. Your support has provided me with much of the motivation to write my third volume. This time I will explore in more depth the stories of some of my patients, alongside subjects such as the coronavirus pandemic, personal observations and life experiences.

I would also like to thank my friends, family and the writers' club for their continued help and advice; my staff and patients for the inspiration they have given me, and I would like to extend a special thanks to my very helpful publisher, Jim Bruce (www.ebooklover.co.uk).

Although the stories are very much true, I have changed the names and some identifiable details for the sake of confidentiality.

I very much hope you enjoy reading these stories as much as I enjoyed writing them.

Dr M A Moss

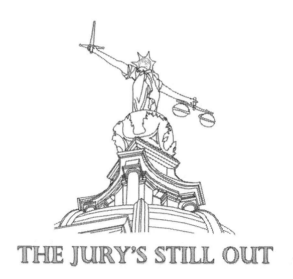

THE JURY'S STILL OUT

Chapter 1

The scene: the famous Central Criminal Court, known as The Old Bailey, London.
Date: Friday, March 27, 2020.

In front of the court a crowd of journalists were jostling each other, including some familiar faces of TV reporters from the BBC, ITV, Sky news and many others. They eagerly awaited a very high-profile cargo coming to the court.

Suddenly the crowd saw a glimpse of the convoy, and all were concentrated on the fast procession of police cars, with their flashing blue lights and blaring sirens. Soon the journalists located the notorious big white van and photographers, with many flashes, rushed to get a photo through the thick dark glass windows of the very secure van.

Someone in the crowd shouted, "We got the b***** at last!" Another shouted, "Allah Akbar!" (God is great), while another called out, "Hallelujah!"

Many policemen in fluorescent protective gear, surrounded by armed officers, rushed to the doors of the court, carrying the accused in a big tightly sealed glass box. They placed the box behind a well-positioned powerful microphone, then swiftly left the area and sat in the court hall, awaiting instructions.

Inside the courtroom there were many people – young and old – and the public gallery above was full. The 12 jurors were in their designated area, all of different genders, varied ages, levels of education and varied experiences in life. They waited nervously for the trial to begin. It was known that there was a bank manager, a single mum (of a school-aged boy), a sociologist, an environmental activist, a senior nurse, a mother of a teenager (who had sadly been fatally stabbed in London in broad daylight), a betting shop worker, an Underground operational manager, a civil servant, a retired teacher and a mother of a soldier killed in Iraq.

Court Number 1, Friday, 10:30am

With an atmosphere full of apprehension and anticipation mixed with excitement, the court crier shouted, "All rise!", then sat facing the courtroom beside the court clerk.

In attendance were the Judge, Lord Justice Morrison QC; Prosecution barrister, Mr Flanagan QC; and the accused, Covid-19.

Dr Moss, a GP in south-east London, testified to the accusation that Covid-19 was a serial killer, as it had taken the life of one of his patients, and many others all over the country. Dr Moss's patient was Mr Trent, a 70-year-old retired Army general with underlying health conditions, including diabetes. Dr Moss and his staff had faced great anxiety and distress as they had dealt with Mr Trent just before they'd heard about Covid-19. As that time they had worked with no protective equipment.

The prosecution barrister revealed that Covid-19 had killed and intended to kill thousands, and called for the maximum penalty of multiple life sentences.

Covid-19, with no legal representative, had decided to defend itself.

Lord Justice Morrison asked the accused, "Your name, your age, your occupation and your address."

The accused answered, "My name is Covid-19, famous by the nickname of Coronavirus. My age is a few months, my occupation is a virus, and some people liked to call me 'The Chinese virus' because I was first discovered in China. But I'm not Chinese; I'm a citizen of the world. My previous address was a secret experimental laboratory, but I can't reveal where, as it is a 'matter of national security', as you usually call it. However, I'm free now, you could say I'm sofa-surfing with no fixed abode."

The judge announced, "The charges against you are that you are a serial killer and have committed many crimes against humanity. You have caused extreme anxiety for Dr Moss, his team and many others all over the world. You have separated people by self-isolation from their loved ones and colleagues. You have caused some of them to depart from this earth with no funeral. You have also caused huge economic and financial loss to many people."

Then he asked the question all had waited for: "Do you plead guilty or not guilty?"

Covid-19 replied emphatically, "Not guilty, your honour."

The defendant continued, "In fact I did what I had to do as a matter of necessity, as I had to survive and reproduce, like any other species. Yes, I had to infect some mammals and humans, however I didn't intend to cause harm and I apologise that harm was sometimes done. If you consider me a friend for a little while, then some people might call this harm 'friendly fire' or 'collateral damage', like what happens during a war when some innocent people are injured or killed unintentionally. I've never seen anybody brought to trial for that.

"I tried very hard to avoid harming the children – not like some people all over the world, killing children by different ways and hardly ever facing justice.

"Some people jokingly called me a lady virus, as I stopped sporting events, including football, I made the pubs, coffee shops and betting shops close and I harmed men more than women. But is that perhaps due to hygiene-related bad habits or because men smoke more than women and are more susceptible to my infection? I'm not really sure.

"Look, your Honour and the respected members of the jury, let me explain something to you. I don't lie, I don't steal, and I don't have a bias. I feel that I'm just a scapegoat. You could have directed these accusations at the people who created me and mutated me in the lab, instead of putting me on trial for this crime when I'm just following my natural instincts, doing what I was created to do. But I know you can't and you wouldn't. Your hands are also tied.

"I admit I caused great economic and financial loss, however you may like to consider some mitigating factors in my case. As humans are the ones who created me, I have no mental capacity to make a conscious decision to commit what I did. As I said, you might instead consider my actions as the basic instinct to survive, almost an act of self-defence. Nobody calls a lion a murderer when he kills to survive. Am I so different then? I would go so far as to suggest to you that I'm not guilty by the reasons of diminished responsibility."

Covid-19 paused and in the hushed courtroom it seemed the onlookers started thinking about what had been said.

The judge nodded and Covid-19 continued, "You may remember the credit crunch and the financial disaster that was caused by the greed of the banking sector in 2008? In that case many bank executives took their bonuses of millions while innocent people were made homeless because of these bankers' irresponsible actions. Being homeless means being very vulnerable, as they now couldn't follow the advice of the government to stay at home and stay safe. They had been left in the streets, relying on the kindness of strangers for a sandwich or some food for their pet, if they had one. I haven't seen anybody summoned to court for this injustice like me.

"Haven't you noticed that for the first time in history the famous hotels have opened their doors to thousands of homeless in the streets of the wealthy city of London? Who made that happen? Poor little me – a tiny little invisible virus. Not some grand politician or celebrity.

"Isn't it nice when you ask a single mother about the opportunity to spend time with her child, home educating, and how the child is delighted to be off school. There is no bullying, no governmental targets for teachers with lots of box-ticking and achievement targets, with little energy left to educate the kids. The poor teachers have repeatedly complained, but it fell on deaf ears. There is healthy food at home, instead of crisps with preservatives and artificial colouring, causing the kids to go hyperactive, with so many of them incorrectly labelled as having some unproven fancy disorders. Isn't it nice for them to have time with their mothers to understand each other better? In some homes fathers are able to play with their kids and read them stories – something that sociologists have been trying to under-stand for years; why we've lost that sense of social cohesion, family ties and values? And why some family members communicate with each other using mobile phones while being in the same house?

"People in one street now start knocking on the door of a 90-year-old person living alone to offer him or her a smile and reassurance that they are not alone, despite having no family members around. Thousands of volunteers help the vulnerable and elderly in society, one of the aspects of this pandemic which can reflect positively on wider society, something you should be proud of.

"Environmental activists have for years been highlighting the air pollution caused by the aviation industry, and pollution in our cities because of cars. Many people are now working from home, proving that there is no need to travel all the way to work. The majority of people adhered to the advice to stay at home unless it was "essential", a word which has been a bit elastic, as some people in America went outside to buy guns and marijuana, considering it necessary. They were in long queues observing the social distancing of two metres though!

"Look what has happened now; the sky is blue, the air in London is of better quality, the birds are singing happily and the fish have returned to the less polluted waters of Venice.

"True heroes of our society appeared in the form of nurses and their health care colleagues, who worked tirelessly, looking after sick people despite the lack of testing facilities and protective equipment, which they badly needed. Instead they got a lot of conferences and meetings with representatives parroting the repeated vague and empty promises by the politicians, who instructed their administrations, with their bureaucratic machinery of the health system, who in turn sent plenty of guidelines, urgent messages, protocols and pathways, with hundreds of pages filled with many charts, drawings and diagrams. These kept everybody in the health profession reading day and night until they got headaches and were not sure whether it was from the infection or the actions of the government!

"When protective equipment was given, some health care professionals commented that it was only good for making sandwiches, as it was substandard, according to the World Health Organisation. Equipment also came too late, as the Chinese gave the world a clear warning, with ample time to react.

"For the first time we witnessed even the most arrogant and ignorant politicians and world leaders listening humbly to doctors and scientists, who were previously under-appreciated in society at the expenses of some of the celebrities, surrounded by their halos of false fame.

"London is much quieter now, with fewer gatherings, no more gangs in the streets, with fewer stabbings, after being like an endemic disease in the capital, with police struggling with staff shortages.

"Some people may argue that domestic violence may go up due to isolation and high levels of stress, especially as men have no football to watch and no pubs to go to. Arguments between partners may increase – if they are self-employed they may stop working and the financial pressure may be mounting. But all this is no fault of mine.

"I agree that betting shops are closed, but you know very well what having a gambling addiction does to people. If you don't then, please ask Dr Moss and his team.

"I like your invention of the phrase 'gamble responsibly'. I think the punters will find other ways, like online gambling, instead of going to the betting shops for the time being. I did my best, and the rest is up to you guys.

"Look at what happened in the Underground; everyone behaving very civilised, with few people in the carriages, all trying their best to apply the rule of two metres social distancing. Where are the days gone by, when commuters repeatedly complained about the very crowded carriages – some people called them cattle trucks. An apology is due here to the cattle and the animal welfare organisations.

"May I remind you that the word honesty in the dictionary is hardly applied nowadays? Look at some countries, which initially refused to admit the coronavirus illness and recorded many deaths as other causes, like heart attacks and other illnesses, fearing for their incomes and the economy. But the minute the United Nations announced the provision of billions of dollars to help the affected countries, many started to readily announce their coronavirus deaths! I hope the money will go into the right pockets this time, and you know what I mean.

"I wonder about the hypocrisy, false virtues, avarice and greed that some world leaders encourage. They support fighting between tribes and countries all over the world for any trivial and unconvincing reasons; they sell their arms, claiming that they create jobs for their citizens and fill their pockets with blood money. It doesn't matter how many people are killed in these wars, or what the colour of the money is. Then they encourage money laundering and tax havens. Let me just remind you that I'm a virus and I don't have rockets, guns, cluster bombs or nuclear weapons to cause havoc with.

"I heard somebody in this court talking about the damages I should pay to the victims. Let me declare that I'm a weak and poor virus; I can't afford to pay a single penny. You may like to ask whoever created me in the laboratories, however I advise you not to waste your time, as everybody will deny any relationship with me, and they will wait for the issue to die down, like many others in history, then they can claim a victory of some sort, as they always do. They never learn!

"And as long as we are talking about money, I'd like to remind Dr Moss and his colleagues, who were screaming to the politicians and top managers for years about the lack of funding for the poor NHS, and whose words fell on deaf ears as usual, that during this pandemic the money has surprisingly come from every direction. It is because of me that an assessment and a real evaluation of the health system everywhere has been done, and it revealed that some organisations were not supplied with adequate levels of equipment to face a pandemic like this. You are welcome, Dr Moss.

"I heard another talking about a conspiracy theory that I was created to get rid of the 'useless eaters', as described by some American politician a number of years ago. By 'useless eaters', he meant the elderly citizens who are a burden on the economy – it seems some governments and some politicians now think the same way. But I can't really comment on this.

"Let me remind you that I heard some religious leaders in your society describing me to be 'a warning from God' – if you believe in one – as you have exceeded the limits of greed and extravagance in this land of plenty, a land in which people throw away food which is sufficient to feed a complete hungry nation somewhere else in the world. In this ordeal, people realised that in some situations in life, money, which is considered to be a 'God' for some people, has little value apart from buying toilet paper, hand sanitisers and anti-bacterial wipes; it can't buy souls back. Death became a grim reality in many people's minds, and many reflected on the only power of their mighty God.

"And finally, please let me remind you that I'm not a racist, like some people. I don't discriminate between races, religions, the colour of the skin, the shape of the eyes. There is no difference between the poorest and the wealthiest, the unemployed and the highly paid, a prime pickpocket and a prime minster, a commoner and a member of a royal family.

"May I offer my sincere apologies for any inconvenience I have caused to anyone, and I hope you have learned a few comprehensive lessons of humanity; that very precious word which elevates you higher and higher than the rest of the species.

"I hope that you consider my position, and I trust that many of you will have a strong conscience to offer me a fair trial."

Silence and anticipation filled the court. Everyone was bewildered by what they had heard from Covid-19.

Suddenly the judge announced, "Court adjourned!"

And the jury's still out.

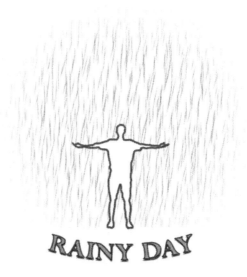

RAINY DAY

Chapter 2

We sometimes face tough, challenging days at the surgery, when you end up tearing out your hair, swearing heavily, with smoke billowing from your ears. But this particular Monday was one of the worst.

I started the day as usual with a positive attitude, taking the short drive from home to the clinic, usually around 25 minutes, and aiming to be half-an-hour early for my morning session.

I wanted to prepare for the day ahead, sorting some patients' test results and writing a few urgent letters before I started the morning session – or the "moaning session", as some of my colleagues call it.

It was raining heavily with strong winds, and I forgot to take an umbrella. I was just back from a short sunny break abroad, facing the reality of grim English weather.

Listening to the radio, I drove through a deep puddle at the side of the road and suddenly the dashboard lights went haywire, flashing orange, yellow, red, with warning messages I couldn't read. Then the engine cut out.

I pulled over and switched on the hazard flashers. I decided not to call the breakdown service but to ring my son Adam, who knows more about my car than I do. He thought it might be a computer hitch and advised me to switch off everything and try to start the car after a few minutes. Surprisingly, it worked.

I continued my journey on the waterlogged road, but unfortunately there was an accident. A motorbike had hit an oncoming car; the car behind the bike tried to stop to avoid hitting the bike and caused multiple collisions. There were two ambulances and three police cars at the scene and traffic was being diverted, which made me late for work.

Arriving at the clinic entrance the smell of chemical cleaner and a hint of excrement hit my nose. Our enthusiastic receptionist Liz was scrubbing the entrance mat and explained that it had been smeared with dog poo from the bottom of someone's shoe.

"It's a dirty job, but somebody has to do it," she told me cheerily.

I entered the crowded reception, with patients waiting for the nurses and some coming in early for my session. I greeted them all with the usual "good morning". I recognised the familiar face of a young patient, John Marshall, whose face said it all: "What's good about it?"

Heading to my den – I mean the consultation room – Kate, one of our receptionists, stopped me, waving an urgent request from one of our locums for an urgent referral. A patient was not happy with a particular hospital and wanted to go to another one. When the locum tried to contact the patient to see which hospital she preferred, she didn't answer her phone.

I rang her later and she answered, apologising that she was busy shopping. I questioned her mobility, as she had requested hospital transport and she was young and relatively healthy.

"Well, I pay my taxes and this transport service is free on the NHS, so why can't I use it?" she demanded. I was in no mood to argue, so I asked her to negotiate that with the hospital transport organisers.

Then I remembered that this young lady used to go to Accident & Emergency on a daily basis for an arm wound sustained while gardening. An A&E consultant had asked her why she didn't go to our surgery for treatment, as A&E was under a lot of pressure and short staffed. "The hospital is nearer," she replied.

Back at my consultation room, Veronica, our senior admin, collared me. "Sorry to bother you, but the practice manager is at a study day, and the deputy is on sick leave. What do you want me to do with this new registration? This patient has two dates of birth," she said.

I looked at the paperwork on this patient, with a long African name. I recalled similar patients with two names, two passports, two driving licences – and even two wives. As a GP it sometimes felt as if we were deputies for the UK Border Force, or an extension of the Home Office.

One day one of our staff found a purse in the street, containing two driving licences for the same lady, with two different names.

I advised Veronica to ask the patient to clarify their real date of birth, as in their passport, and sign a declaration to keep on record. "Good luck!" I told her.

All set to begin the day's consultations, I switched on my computer. We have many layers of securities, with many passwords, and a note appeared, asking me to enter my user name and password. I entered the user name, and I tried hard to remember the password after my holiday. Thankfully, I kept it written in a secure drawer – against the NHS protocol.

However, I was asked to change my password (it does that every short period for security reasons). After I had exhausted all the names of the kids, the wife, the cat, the car, the neighbours and their dog, a new password was finally accepted, despite it being a swear word!

Not in the mood to check patients' blood results and other tests, or the letters in my tray, or even emails, I started the morning consultations very late.

I buzzed for the gloomy John Marshall, but the electronic board in reception wasn't working, so I had to head out to reception and ask for him. I apologised to him for the delay and ushered him into my room. He mumbled something inaudible.

His untidy, grubby appearance and dirty fingernails grabbed my attention, along with the very strong smell of body odour, stale alcohol and cigarettes, all invading my personal space.

"How can I help, John?" I asked.

"Doc, I need my sick note for the Job Centre, as these people have no consideration to my condition and they've stopped my benefits. I'm appealing to them that I can't work."

I interrupted John, saying, "Ah, you can't work at the moment, but you are young, and with some rehabilitation and support, if you are willing, things can go back to a nearly normal life."

"Yes, Doc, I'm trying my best. I've reduced my drinking from ten pints a day to eight or nine. But I'm paying a lot of bills, and a friend in the pub told me that as long as I have dry skin, some doctors call it eczema, and I use water a lot, then I can apply for lower rates for water bills. Can I apply for that, Doc?"

I frowned and replied, "Yes, you can, John. Bring the forms to me and I will see how I can help you." I handed John his sick note, and after he left I sprayed the room with air freshener.

* * * * *

I called for the next patient, named Man Maya Limbu, who was suffering from a bad cough, according to my patient list on the computer screen.

I expected to see a male patient, but it was Mrs Man Limbu, a Nepalese lady in her early fifties, wearing a traditional, colourful Nepalese dress and a heavy dark pink coat.

She looked well and was accompanied by her husband, whom I later learned was an ex-Ghurkha soldier (Nepalese served in the British Army). He was wearing a sporty tracksuit under a long waterproof coat, and was also in his early fifties.

They were new faces to me, as new patients. I introduced myself and greeted them with the only word I know in Nepalese – "Namaste".

Mrs Limbu didn't speak much English so her husband took control and translated for her. "She is not well. Cough, cough," he said.

I asked, "How long has it been, and is it a dry cough or with phlegm?"

Mr Limbu translated for his wife and I was expecting a quick answer. But they discussed it for ages and eventually Mr Limbu answered, "Dry cough for three days."

"Is there a sore throat or anything else?" I asked. Their long discussion continued until finally Mr Limbu replied, "No sore throat."

"OK, any fever?" I asked. They started debating this, yet again, and time was running out on the 10-minute appointment. So I asked for permission to examine the patient.

I swiftly checked her temperature (normal), throat (normal), chest (normal) and heart (normal). I diagnosed a viral infection and advised some simple pain relief if needed, and a soothing honey, lemon and ginger drink to make at home, and gave them a leaflet on how to prepare it.

Mr Limbu replied, "Antibiotics. She wants antibiotics."

"No need for antibiotics," I said.

"But she had this last year and the doctor gave her antibiotics."

"Your wife has a viral infection and antibiotics don't work for a virus. She is fit and healthy and she should be able to clear this infection in few days. If her condition gets worse, you can come back to see me."

But the consultation wasn't over, and Mr Limbu launched into the next point on his agenda.

"You see, doctor, she had a shoulder pain two weeks ago and the GP advised painkiller tablets and said he would refer her to physiotherapy. But we didn't hear from physiotherapy."

I explained that, according to her patient record, the referral had been sent but it would take a little time as the service was under pressure. I gave him a leaflet with exercises which Mrs Limbu could do at home.

Then he showed me some pink anti-inflammatory tablets and said, "She only took one tablet but felt dizzy, with a headache, and stopped taking them." He produced a pharmacy receipt and asked, "Can we get a refund for the rest of the tablets?" I told him to ask the pharmacy about that.

"One last thing doctor; a sick certificate for one week off work."

I asked what work she did, and he replied, "She doesn't work."

"So why does she need a sick certificate?"

"No, it's not for her, doctor, it's for me. I work as a security guard but she is very ill and I want one week off work to look after her."

"Well, I'll give her the sick note, and you can take it to your employer to give you some time off, if they are happy to do so. Good luck then."

Mr Limbu took a tissue from the tissue box on the desk, passed it to his wife, then took another one for himself and put it in his pocket (some people might say "one for the road", I suppose).

He then asked if they could weigh themselves on the scales in the corner of the room, and I reluctantly nodded in agreement while writing up her notes.

They started taking off their coats, taking out a wallet and keys, and removing their shoes (while I watched patiently). I then spotted a computer reminder that Mrs Limbu needed a smear test with the nurse, so I mentioned this to Mr Limbu.

He didn't seem to understand and answered, "Can I have one as well?"

I explained that a smear test was for ladies only, and added that I'd ask a Nepalese doctor working with us to contact them to explain more.

Mr Limbu then commented that his wife had put on one kilo in weight. I recorded her weight and noticed she had no record of smoking, so I asked Mr Limbu, "Does she smoke?"

"No, she doesn't smoke – but she chews tobacco."

I was in a quandary, as patient records only have boxes to tick for smoker, non-smoker, or ex-smoker. I decided to list her as "non-smoker – who chews tobacco".

With that, the couple finally left, after over-running their 10-minute appointment by many minutes. As all GPs know, that's life!

* * * * *

Before I buzzed for the next patient, the phone rang. It was Kate, from reception. "Sorry, doctor, Andrew from the Coroner's Office is on the line. He wants to talk to you about one of our patients."

"Hello, Andrew, how can I help?" I asked.

"Dr Moss, the Coroner's Office had been informed about the sudden death of Mrs Sallow in her sleep. Her husband told us that she had asthma and last year had a small heart attack. Is that right?"

I answered yes, and Andrew asked if I could issue a death certificate for her. I said I would quickly review her patient record.

"I last saw her two months ago, when she had poor sleep due to family problems and repeated rows with her daughter and her husband about financial issues. I gave her sleeping tablets for one week, and I've not seen her since. However, another script of sleeping tablets was issued three days ago and repeated again after two days, as it was reported as lost on a bus. I think in these circumstances, and according to the rules, she was not seen by me or other colleagues within 14 days, I doubt if I can say for sure the cause of death, and I have to leave this matter with you."

Andrew replied, "That is fine, thank you, Doc."

* * * * *

I checked the time and, as expected, I was now running a bit late and as the digital board was still not working I had to walk to the reception to call my next patient.

Along the corridor leading to the reception hall and office, I heard a loud voice, getting louder. "I want to see the practice manager, or I'll write a complaint. How dare that doctor keep looking at my boobs!"

I was about to go back to my room, but I realised that the practice manager was not around.

We do encourage constructive criticism, as it helps to improve our service, but we try to avoid written complaints, which mean the parties involved write statements, meetings are held and there's a lot of very unnecessary bureaucracy.

I kept my head down and entered the reception office, where Liz briefed me about Ruth Smith's complaint. She had come in for her regular sick note to take to the Job Centre, and was added to the end of Dr Dikko's list.

He decided to examine her back to justify the sick note, especially as she'd had recent investigations, which were all normal. Ruth refused bluntly and he had to accept it. She asked him to back-date the certificate from the previous week, but he said that he could only give it from today, so Ruth raged at him and came blustering into reception.

I've known Dr Dikko for years; he is happily married, he is a granddad, he is trustworthy. He is retired officially, but we asked for his kind help in a few sessions to ease the pressure due to the shortage of doctors nationwide. Many junior doctors have decided to work overseas for higher salaries, a better working environment, and a better lifestyle. Who can blame them?

I've known Ruth Smith since the day she registered with us. When I was reviewing her registration documents, I noticed that she was a young lady, recently moved to our area, and registered with her four-year-old son. She was a single mum, with a few health problems. She wrote in the 'family history' section: depression, drugs, assault, rape, asthma, diabetes, alcoholism, liver disease. She wrote in the 'occupation' section: ex-gang affiliation.

So I decided to calm Ruth down, offering her a few minutes in my room, and I asked Liz to apologise to my next patients for the delay.

Ruth repeated what Liz had told me, and I explained to her why doctors had to examine patients, especially if they were not familiar with their case.

"As you refused to be examined, Dr Dikko accepted that, and he will document it in your record. And the point about him refusing to give you a back-dated sick note, it is a courtesy of the doctor," I told her.

"I give you a sick note because I know you and I'm aware that you will get a medical check by the benefits team. Don't forget this protocol came after the Job Centre wrote to us that a fellow had reported that his mate was in Ibiza in Spain at the same time that he had a back-dated sick note. That guy posted his good time in Ibiza on Facebook, and it was in the local paper a few months ago."

Ruth nodded in agreement, then came to the sticky question. Was the decent Dr Dikko really looking at her boobs? With a guilty look, she replied, "I have no money, doctor, and there were no appointments with you, unless I waited a week or two."

I stopped her to say, "Well, this is a nationwide problem. However, I was asking you about the boob thing." She didn't respond, so I think I got the message from her silence.

I asked her to tell Liz to put her down as an additional appointment on one of my sessions the following week and said farewell to her.

I just kept thinking, 'thank God I know my patients'. I imagined that if somebody mischievously wrote to our regulatory body the GMC (General Medical Council), they would be delighted to flex their muscles, sharpen their teeth, and get down to some serious business, only to find at the end that it was just a false allegation, after the damage had been done.

* * * * *

After a few seconds of reflection, the beep of the digital board signalled that my next patient had been called. It seems it had started working again. The door opened, I smiled and said "Hello, Obioma."

I've know Obioma for years, since she came to Britain, and we had agreed that I called her by her first name, as her surname is very long and I might mispronounce it.

Obioma is a friendly and charming young lady in her mid-forties, short and stout, with curly hair and glasses. She wears very colourful clothes.

She had reported chronic lower back pain, which had been investigated before and everything was fine. But she continued to complain of the on-and-off pain.

She uses a walking stick sporadically, when needed. On one visit to the surgery she was using her stick, but the following day I spotted her dashing to catch a bus in the main street, with no sign of her walking aid.

On her last visit, Obioma received a note to give to the university where she was studying, as she couldn't attend courses or sit examinations because of her bad back.

She already had an extension to her visa, so there was no need for her to study any more, I supposed.

And how about the loan she took out for the study? Ah, the continuous sick note might cover that. She wouldn't be able to work to repay the debt because of her continuous depression and she was on medication.

It made me wonder if some patients actually took the medication, or was it just for the documentation that they were on medication. They keep asking for it, but do they really take it? Who knows?

Obioma taught me a few things during the years of consultations. She knew of more than one illegal immigrant who worked for the Home Office, not necessarily as an official but working with subcontractors, like cleaners.

"OK, how can I help you today, Obioma?" I asked.

"I feel very tired, I have the shivers and feel hot then cold for two to three days since I came back from Africa."

I looked at her notes and saw that she'd been prescribed malaria tablets before her travels.

"Did you take the course of malaria tablets?"

She looked guilty. "No, Doc, I forgot. I thought it was free on the NHS but it wasn't and it was expensive."

"You could have had over-the-counter anti-malarial. It works out cheaper," I replied.

"Do you think it is malaria, Doc?"

"I'm sending you to the hospital to confirm it with a blood test, and next time you go to Africa, take your malaria tablets, please."

I couldn't resist asking her, "By the way, did you take the walking stick and the depression tablets with you to Africa, or did you forget them as well?"

"No, Doc, I didn't take the walking stick or the depression tablets, as I don't get back pain or depression in Africa!"

I thought the consultation had finished, but Obioma added, "You referred me to the hospital two months ago for my tummy problem, you remember? Well, I'm sorry but I missed the appointment as I was in Africa."

I asked her, "Did you mention that you were going to Africa so I could have conveyed it to the hospital?"

"No, Doc, I forgot!"

"OK, you can ring the appointment number to send you another appointment."

"Your receptionist advised me to do that, but when I rang the appointment office they insisted that I go back to the GP for another referral."

"OK, Obioma, I'll ask one of our staff to request another appointment for you … and this time remember not to forget it!" I told her, as she shuffled out of the room, looking guilty.

* * * * *

My next patient on that mad morning was Maria, who was suffering from ankle pain. I've know Maria – in her 30s, small and elegant, with short blonde hair – since she first came to England from Eastern Europe.

On her very first appointment she was accompanied by a friend from her home country to act as translator, as Maria had difficulties with English. Before we began, Maria handed me a small brown envelope, which I expected might contain a request for something, or a script from her home country for medication.

I was stunned to find a crisp £50 note inside the envelope.

The translator said, "It's for you, doctor. We do that in our country."

I smiled and explained politely that we don't do that in England; we just do our duties and are paid to do so.

This day Maria had come in for the results of an X-ray taken a week earlier after she twisted her ankle during her work as a cleaner. She also needed a sick note and more pain relief, as she still had swelling and pain.

While I was typing up her notes, she handed me a two-page form. I gathered that after she'd had the X-ray, the hospital staff had given her a feedback form. She'd asked them for help to fill it in, but they said they were short-staffed and she should take it to her GP.

I looked at the survey form but I didn't want to spend valuable time filling it in for her and holding up my other patients waiting to see me.

So I called for the ever helpful Veronica, our senior administrator. I introduced her to Maria, explained the situation and handed her the form.

Maria looked relieved and grateful, but there was a different message in Veronica's big brown eyes and her facial expression!

At our staff meeting a few weeks earlier, Veronica had brought to my attention a few articles she'd taken from the internet and newspapers, where the Health Secretary had pledged to cut bureaucracy, which cost the NHS a lot of money. It was an empty promise, of course.

"Good luck, Veronica, with a smile of course!" was all I could say to her now as she glared at me, no doubt festering about yet more NHS form-filling and red tape.

* * * * *

My next patient was Mrs Jacob, in her late fifties, very hard-working, elegant and well educated. I've known her for years and she always looks younger than her age. Sadly, she'd recently lost her husband after a long battle with cancer.

Her appointment was for arthritis and blood pressure issues, and she was looking tired and sad, as if she hadn't slept for few days. I understood this as she was still grieving the loss of her husband.

"The arthritis in my knee and wrist is getting worse but this is not the issue," she told me. "The issue is, I'm still under treatment, but I would like to go back and do light work, as I was made redundant by the company before my husband died."

Mrs Jacob then told me that she'd written a letter of complaint, with the help of her daughter as her wrist was swollen, to the manager of her local Job Centre about her treatment there by staff.

Mrs Jacob handed me a copy of it to read. She started crying and I consoled her, offering her some tissues.

I glanced quickly at the letter and my attention was drawn to a sentence about a young assessor shouting at Mrs Jacob in front of other jobless people at the centre.

Mrs Jacob had been accused of arriving half-an-hour late for her appointment at the centre, when in fact she had been 30 minutes early. The assessor stormed off, telling Mrs Jacob to wait.

A security guard who heard the shouting thought Mrs Jacob had been causing trouble, so he came over and stood menacingly behind her.

The assessor returned, shouting again, and said "Show me your job search record."

Mrs Jacob replied, "I'm sorry, I wasn't able to apply for jobs as my wrist is swollen, as you can see. A letter from GP – here is a copy – says I'm still grieving the death of my husband. And I'm still under treatment for the flare-up of arthritis."

Then another assessor came over to tell Mrs Jacob there had been a mix-up with another Mrs Jacob, who had actually arrived late, and apologised to her.

In her letter, Mrs Jacob added, "It was all too late. I burst in tears. I couldn't take any more of that attitude, and I left the place without signing on. I'd never felt so humiliated in my life. The assessor was very aggressive and assumed that I was late, which was inaccurate. There was no apology from her, it was from the other older and more experienced assessor."

I realised that this experience had caused her stress and poor sleep, and no doubt this had affected her blood pressure, which was high.

I sympathised with her, calmed her down, reviewed her medications, gave her a leaflet about sleep hygiene and an extension of her sick note, and advised her to get some over-the-counter medication from the pharmacy to help her sleep.

"Thanks, doctor," she said as she left the room.

* * * * *

Before I called my next patient, Kate from reception knocked on my door, asking if I could help Dr Newman next door for a second opinion.

I went in to find a patient, Mr Rosen, sitting calmly in her room. She looked more distressed than him.

"How can I help?" I asked.

Dr Newman explained that Mr Rosen had requested cream for eczema, which he'd had few years earlier, which also helped with his erections.

He'd also requested a test for the level of his mother's milk in his urine, as requested by a martial arts team he wanted to join! What the devil was he talking about?

Dr Newman had tried to explain repeatedly that there was no such thing as a cream for eczema that also boosted erections.

But Mr Rosen kept arguing, saying, "Please, look at my record. Dr Moss gave it to me before, but I can't remember when."

I asked Mr Rosen, "Are you taking your medication regularly?" He gave an emphatic 'yes'. I looked at his record on the computer, and he was correct.

I said, "Show me the eczema then." He showed me his arms and I pointed out a small area of dry skin.

"That's fine, Mr Rosen, we will prescribe you the cream for that, the same cream you had in the past, to use for one week only, as we agreed before," I told him.

He thanked me and, to the surprise of Dr Newman, I reached for her computer mouse and pointed the arrow on the screen to the list of Mr Rosen's problems, which showed mental illness, and in the medication section his anti-psychotic drugs.

Dr Newman nodded in acknowledgement.

I prescribed a mild steroid cream, once daily for one week, and did a urine test request form, and gave Mr Rosen a urine pot to bring when he was ready, explaining that it might take some days to process the request.

Mr Rosen smiled, thanked us and left, while Dr Newman stared at me in disbelief.

I explained to her that when Mr Rosen first visited the surgery, about six years earlier, his initial consultations were fine. But then he asked for a cream he said he'd been using for 20 years – although there was no record on this. He added that he was waiting for permission to join a martial arts team, on the condition that the level of mother's milk in his urine was tested.

I had called his psychiatric consultant about these issues, and we agreed that he was generally stable, but had brief delusional episodes, which usually disappeared after two or three days, as long as he was taking his medication.

"Since then, every few years, as documented in his record, he gets a small tube of the cream and a request for the urine test, which is never sent to the lab. Over the next few days he forgets all about it," I told Dr Newman.

"Have a nice day, Dr Newman," I smiled.

* * * * *

Back in my consulting room, my next patient was Melissa, aged five, who was with her mother. I've known Melissa since she was a baby.

Melissa was very popular with the reception staff, as she always asked them on every visit, "I want to see the goodest doctor!"

She was suffering from a fever and a sore throat for two days, the same recurrent tonsillitis she had four or five times a year.

I remembered I had referred her about two months earlier for a surgical opinion, as her condition was getting worse. It affected her school attendance, and now the school was asking for a letter of proof every time she visited the surgery.

This was something our professional organisations asked us not to provide to schools, as the administrative workload was beyond belief.

I prescribed antibiotics and advised Melissa's mother to photocopy the prescription as proof of attendance at the surgery.

The mother asked, "Why does it take so long for the ear, nose and throat appointment to come through?"

I explained the local protocols, guidelines and criteria for accepting referrals, and the pressure on the NHS in dealing with a lot of very complex cases and cancer priorities. I reassured her that she would get an appointment in due course.

But the mother wasn't happy and vowed to write to the hospital complaining about the delay.

It left me with an uneasy feeling that due to the increased pressure on the ailing NHS, we can't please everyone all of the time.

* * * * *

Before I called the next patient, I received an urgent message from a probation officer, asking for information on one of our patients, named Jordan.

I called the probation officer, who said Jordan hadn't signed with them on two occasions, as he should have done, and mentioned he was not well and had been seen at the surgery during that period.

"Jordan has marks of old self-harm, and feels very low, but with no suicidal thoughts," he said.

I said there was no record that Jordan had visited the surgery in the past three months, and obviously he'd stopped taking his anti-depressant.

"You'd better send him to our surgery to be assessed urgently," I added. He thanked me, and the call ended.

Suddenly, a screen message appeared, saying, "The hospital rat rang, enquiring about Mr J. Bond, DOB 1/4/1941, please ring extension 007 when you have a minute."

James Bond? 007? Was this a practical joke? We didn't have any patients who were 'licensed to kill'. As for rats, I do remember seeing some in the London hospitals where I used to work, but I wasn't sure why they would be calling me.

I was baffled and decided to ring the receptionist Liz, who wrote the message, bearing in mind that we, as a team, sometimes play jokes on each other to relieve some of the intense pressure of NHS work.

"Hello Liz, I've read your message. Did they say which rat in which hospital, as there are many of them?"

She laughed and replied, "No, they said the doctor knows. But I have to admit I couldn't get the long surname of the lady who contacted us, as she said it very quickly."

"OK, Liz, leave it with me to sort that rat out."

I typed in the date of birth of the patient. It was Mr Jeffery Bond, a new patient to our surgery, explaining why his name didn't ring a bell. Mr Bond was aged 78, with terminal cancer. He had moved to our area to live with his sister and had a long list of chronic illnesses.

I decided to ring the hospital and followed the instructions of the automated voice, dialling in extension 007. I half-expected a deep voice to answer, "The name's Bond, James Bond."

To my surprise, a female voice answered, "R.A.T. Sister Wikramanayake speaking."

"Hello, Sister, I'm returning your call regarding Mr Bond. But please, before we start, as I'm not good with these new abbreviations, what does RAT stand for?"

"RAT is Rapid Assessment Team," she replied.

The sister mentioned that Mr Bond was stable and had been reviewed by a RAT consultant, but he needed to know what medication Mr Bond was taking, as he had forgotten to bring them with him. I happily gave her all the information she needed.

I then cheekily asked Liz to keep up to date with all the new NHS abbreviations we were bombarded with on a daily basis – RAT, CAT, FAT, HAT and so on.

* * * * *

I was about to finally call my next patient, when there was yet another interruption.

Veronica, our senior admin, appeared at the door to tell me that the nurses' printer had stopped working and one of the reception's computers had crashed. The IT team had promised to attend ASAP, probably within two or three hours.

"Thankfully my computer is still working," I told her. Then the screen went black, but luckily it reconnected again.

Our computer system is very old and unstable, and all its problems have been reported to the NHS Trust. But all we get are political statements and a message, reading between the lines, to carry on. Hopefully one day they may listen.

Suddenly I received a high-priority screen message from Liz, our receptionist.

"Sorry to bother you, but the afternoon locum nurse rang and she can't come in, as her child was very ill and taken to the hospital. We tried to shift the patients, but two of them can't be contacted, as they haven't updated their mobile numbers, and they may turn up. Alisha, the senior nurse, is fully booked, actually over-booked, and the locum doctor doesn't allow extras on his list. So can we put their names under your list as extras, please?"

I rang Liz to agree to her request – and she hit me with another administrative problem.

"Just to keep you informed that Kate, the morning receptionist, has broken her ankle."

Liz was kind enough to cover for Kate for the morning, adding to her huge work load, until the practice manger could sort out the staff rota the following day.

I read the notes for the two extra patients I'd agreed to see.

One of them read bizarrely, "The bum increased in size and needs assessment."

I asked Liz what this was all about. She read it and screamed, "Oh, my God! Sorry, it was meant to be 'a skin tag on the bum increased in size and needs assessment'. But the computer crashed and I didn't notice that the skin tag had been removed. Sorry, sorry!"

* * * * *

My next patient was Mr Thorne, whom I remembered was a difficult person.

When he was new to our surgery, he came to the reception to book an appointment, but there were none left. So he went back home and after a few hours he contacted the surgery, requesting a home visit.

He reluctantly told the receptionist what his problem was and she booked a slot and told him a doctor would phone him.

I was the duty doctor at that time and I saw the message the new receptionist had written: Pain in the neck. I had to correct it for her, as she meant 'neck pain'.

I rang Mr Thorne and discovered he was lying in an awkward position on the sofa, watching TV. I advised some simple pain relief and offered him an appointment the next day to see the duty doctor.

Mr Thorne's name was well-known to our staff and written on his warning window was: Don't book with a certain nurse or certain doctors.

I had dealt with his written complaints about:

A nurse who didn't tell him to press on the cotton wool after she took his blood for testing, caused bleeding from the site and a small bruise on the arm;

A locum doctor who, following the Trust's policy, was reluctant to give him medication he could obtain from any pharmacy over the counter, as he probably noticed the very long list of drug allergies and side-effects on his record;

Another doctor who was less sympathetic and didn't greet him at the beginning of the consultation.

Another time he complained to me verbally when I couldn't find his hospital letter in our record, as the consultant had told Mr Thorne to contact his GP after a week. I explained to Mr Thorne that some hospital letters arrived after 4- 6 weeks, due to the pressure on the NHS, and sometimes even after few months. I had to ring the consultant's secretary, asking her to fax the letter directly to me, to avoid any delay in the post.

I greeted Mr Thorne, who told me, "I'm here to check my blood pressure."

I measured his blood pressure and told him, "Right, it's still high and you remember at the last consultation I explained to you that your record shows repeated high blood pressure readings, and your family history of your father having high blood pressure, and you are still reluctant to start treatment."

He swiftly answered, "Nah, I don't think I have blood pressure. I'm fit as a fiddle."

I replied, "Still, you can be fit but have high blood pressure. It is entirely up to you, we only advise."

"OK, Doc, I told you that I hate medicine, and I want to do it my way by doing exercise and reducing my weight. But I can't at the moment because of my leg ulcer."

"Oh yes, about your leg ulcer. The record shows that you didn't attend our nurse for a dressing, and on many occasions you booked a double appointment, which you didn't attend."

"Yes, Doc. I sometimes attend Accident and Emergency in the local hospital instead, as it is near to my home."

"But Mr Thorne, please note that a leg ulcer is not an accident or an emergency. And by the way, I remember the hospital rang about you as a frequent attendant. If we can help you, please, this is a polite reminder to attend your appointments with our nurses. Now, do you want to start the blood pressure medications?"

"OK then, Doc, and can you give me a sick note from last month as the locum doctor refused to do so, as he doesn't know me, and didn't like to backdate the certificate."

I obliged and he left, however his case hadn't finished yet.

While reading his letters, I noticed a gynaecology letter (women's speciality letter), so I called Veronica and pointed out the gynaecology letter in his record had to be removed and filed in his wife's note, as it had been filed by mistake in his notes.

Luckily, he never knew about that mistake – or I'm sure he would have complained.

* * * * *

I then answered a phone query about a patient's medications allergy, then I had a request to call Mrs Doris Arnold, a 90-year-old, house-bound patient with severe arthritis and very poor mobility. I'd always told her to "ring us if you need anything".

I phoned and she told me, "I'm not well, Doc. I fell from the chair and couldn't get up. Thank God I can reach the phone. Can you send somebody to help me get up to the chair?"

"Did you hurt any part of your body or have any pain anywhere?"

"No, Doc, I just need some help to get up. My carer just left before I fell. I've rung her but she's not answering."

"If I send somebody, you probably would not be able to open the door for them. OK, leave it with me."

I told our staff to try repeatedly to ring the carer and send a text in case she was driving. If there was no answer, they should ring the agent manager to send another carer to help Doris, and let me know the outcome after I returned from my home visits.

Thankfully, after a little while there was a successful outcome and Doris was helped back in her favourite chair.

* * * * *

I grabbed my doctor's bag and ran to the car in the pouring rain, still with no umbrella, to visit 80-year-old Mrs Sparrow, a lovely lady who lived alone and was house-bound.

She had multiple illnesses; knee arthritis, asthma, sigmoid colon diverticular disease, kidney and heart failures, but they were reasonably well controlled by medication. She was supported very well by her daughter, who lived nearby.

Mrs Sparrow had a productive cough for few days, vomited once and felt lethargic with abdominal discomfort. I examined her, took her temperature, pulse and blood pressure, which were fine. There were no signs of heart failure, her abdomen was soft with mild tenderness in the left lower part, most probably from an inflamed colon caused by the diverticular disease.

I explained the options of treatment, and one of them was to be taken to hospital for blood tests, X-rays and antibiotics, with observation by the nurses. She agreed that would be the best option, and she rang her daughter to tell her. The daughter was very happy that her mother would be observed by the nurses, as she lived alone.

I was about to ring for an ambulance, but Mrs Sparrow requested about an hour to prepare herself, and to ring a boiler engineer to cancel his visit in the afternoon.

I called the hospital A&E, informed them about the case, and rang for an ambulance service, telling the controller about Mrs Sparrow's condition and requesting the ambulance in an hour.

"Doctor, you said she had heart failure. I'm afraid the computer picked up the word 'heart' and told me to send a blue-light ambulance at once, which should be with you in minutes," said the controller.

"But Mrs Sparrow is not ready yet. She has a history of heart failure but it is very stable, and there's no need for a blue-light ambulance. I'm here, her doctor, I'm very familiar with her case, and it is my clinical judgement and responsibility. You can save the blue light for very urgent cases," I said.

"Sorry doctor, it is our protocol."

"OK, can you give me your manager, please?"

"Sorry, he's on his lunch break."

I wasn't in the mood for an argument. Then I heard the ambulance siren and the vehicle pulled up in front of the house. The crew asked Mrs Sparrow if she was ready, and she told them, "No, I'll need at least an hour."

They looked at me, so I told them about my conversation with their controller. They called their base and had a heated debate with the controller, saying that Mrs Sparrow was stable, but not ready to go, and that they would return an hour later to pick her up.

* * * * *

Back again in the rain, I drove to a local funeral parlour to view a body and complete the required forms for a cremation.

It's supposed to be a straight-forward procedure, if all parties are happy and there are no concerns of any kind. However, while viewing the body I noticed an old bruise on the side of the head and a smaller one on the chest.

I asked the treating doctor, relatives and the nurses who had looked after him in his last days about these bruises. They said he had been taking Warfarin (blood thinner medication) for an irregular heart beat, which can cause bruising.

However, his death had been expected, due to very extensive cancer with metastasis, and none of the involved staff or relatives had any concerns, so I filled in the forms for everybody to proceed with the cremation.

* * * * *

Back at the surgery car park, I ran to the building to avoid getting soaked by the torrential downpour. But my blue suit ended up covered in dark rain spots.

However, my mood bounced back as I spotted the familiar face of Mrs Richardson, was leaving the surgery and reading her prescription. She smiled at me and was about to say something but noticed I was in a rush.

Passing by reception, Liz saw me and ran out after me.

"Liz, please may I have a banana and a cup of tea, and then you can tell me what you wanted."

Walking together towards the staff room for the cup of tea, I noticed on the table of the meeting room some sandwiches and drinks. In the room were two familiar palliative care nurses, a community heart failure nurse and Veronica, who was looking at me and wanting to say something urgent.

Liz confirmed that they were all waiting for me for a Gold Standard Framework meeting, where we review the termi-nally-ill patients and chart their progress.

"Oh, Liz, Sorry, but I really forgot about this meeting. I remember now that it had been postponed, as I was away last week. But who will see my patients who are waiting now?" I said. Liz said Veronica had already distributed some patients to the locum and the duty doctors.

"The good news is that the IT team came and fixed the nurses' printer and the reception computer. The less good news is that the hospital lab rang to say they are installing new software, which has caused problems for the afternoon results. They are working on it and they will send our results when things are back to normal," said Liz.

At the meeting we progressed through our patients one by one, until we stopped at Mr May, who had diabetes and advanced prostate cancer.

He had sadly passed away, but the local pharmacy kept delivering his medication through his letterbox.

One of our receptionists lived next door to Mr May's daughter and was aware of his death. She brought it to my attention and as I had no documentation confirming his death yet, I decided to ring the pharmacy, who confirmed that the medications had been requested by the patient, or one of his relatives.

I decided to ring the daughter, as next of kin, and kindly asked her to take all his medications back to the pharmacy, and tell them that her dad had died, and there was no need to request the drugs from the surgery any more.

Back at the meeting, I mentioned the sad case of a lady I had just visited. She was in her early 40s, with no previous history of abdominal symptoms. She was last seen six months earlier by a nurse for a routine smear test, which came back normal. She'd also had many blood tests for health checks, and all these were normal.

A few days earlier, the patient noticed swelling and pain in her leg in the evening and went to A&E. Surprisingly, she was diagnosed with DVT (Deep Venous Thrombosis, a clot in the leg).

There were no obvious causes for that clot, but further investigations revealed she had extensive abdominal metastatic cancer. The woman was admitted to hospital to begin urgent chemotherapy.

I was shocked when I received a fax from the hospital informing me about the findings, and when I read that she had been discharged home I added her name to the home visit list.

I mentioned her case at the meeting so that the palliative care team would keep an eye on her.

The meeting ended, and I'd managed to eat my banana – but my cup of tea was stone cold.

* * * * *

Back at my consultation room, I wrote up the home visit before seeing the remaining few patients on my list.

Then came an urgent request from a well-known patient, Mrs Mourad, who was insisting on talking to me only.

I've known Mrs Mourad for years. She would sometimes call the surgery every half-an-hour to see if she could get an appointment for problems such as a mild headache, or sneezing a lot.

Every doctor who dealt with her could see the warning message before seeing her record, with a long list of drug allergies. They had to avoid giving her something she didn't like in the past, so they prescribed something else. Sometimes she said she didn't like pain relief tablets, so she was given capsules instead, and vice versa.

I phoned her and she told me, "Doctor, I have a big problem and I need your help. My daughter and her husband came to visit me last week. They offered to decorate the sitting room, as it is getting very old and the wallpaper is falling off the walls. Well, they have to move the bed from the sitting room – you remember I sleep downstairs now because of my arthritis and I don't go upstairs. Anyway, the bed is very heavy and they can't take it apart, so I rang the council, who decided they can't help. The social services advised me to contact the occupational therapy team in the hospital, who installed the bed in the first place, to help in this matter. So I decided to talk to you about that, for your help."

Thank God she didn't ask me for a home visit to take the bed apart, move it upstairs and reassemble it. Perhaps I could also have put up new wallpaper?

I told her, "I don't mind talking to the occupational health team in the local hospital, but they will take ages to come and do the job for you, as they might be short of staff, or dealing with most urgent cases."

Then I suggested that her son-in-law could just buy some plastic sheeting to cover the bed while he redecorated the room. The bed would not have to be moved upstairs. How about that!

"Yes, doctor, I'll tell him your suggestion."

I never heard back from Mrs Mourad – for a while anyway.

* * * * *

Thank God the next patient, Mr Yusuf, arrived 10 minutes late, making up for my delayed schedule. Glancing at computer screen I noticed he had been booked in for poor sleep. My brain instantly said "fine, quick consultation then", assuming that it'd be something simple.

Mr Yusuf, a young Somali man, in his early 40s, tall and thin, had registered with us only three months earlier and had a very short medical record.

He lived at an address I recognised, down the road from our surgery in a multi-occupancy house belonging to a housing association, which was renting it to the council for temporary dwellers.

I noticed on his problem list: anxiety, depression, post-traumatic stress disorder.

Mr Yusuf entered the room with a house-mate called Mo, acting as translator.

"How is Mr Yusuf?" I asked.

Mo replied, "He is not good, not sleeping. He's had his benefits stopped and he received a letter from the Home Office to sit an English language test."

It transpired that Mr Yusuf had come in the previous week and saw Dr Newman, who gave him a contact number for some counselling.

The counselling service listened to his problems, and gave him the address of the local Citizens Advice Bureau. Mr Yusuf went there early one morning around 7am, waiting in the rain. The staff listened to his problem, through an interpreter, sympathised with him and gave him another number to ring.

Mo rang this number and was surprised to find it was the Immigration Department of the Home Office – who had requested the language test in the first place.

They advised him to contact a GP for supporting letters, which was why they were here to see me.

I was more than happy to support him, and I asked about his sleep.

Mo said, "His poor sleep is because of this letter. Thank God he will be getting it now."

Mo paused for a few seconds and added, "The other problem of sleep is that a new guy from the Far East has joined our house. He used to sleep during the day and pace up and down in the kitchen at night. He took the fire alarm down off the ceiling, alleging that it had a tiny camera spying on us. He cut off the electricity in the main box, as he doesn't want anybody to use the internet, as he believes it has many spies and is controlling him, making him do bad things and sending him messages, driving him mad."

I asked Mo, "Why don't you send this person to us to be seen?"

Mo replied, "He is registered with another surgery far away."

So I advised them to report what they had told me to the housing association, as it had safety issues, and I wished them good luck.

* * * * *

My next patient was Mrs Robertson, in her early 70s, who needed a steroid shoulder injection and other things. With a nice soft Jamaican accent, she was a tall, elegant lady.

I remembered she had retired with her husband to enjoy post-work life, but her husband had been diagnosed with advanced colonic cancer. He battled through a long journey of chemotherapy and radiotherapy, but sadly passed away.

The stress on Mrs Robertson had aged her quickly but she still had a good spirit with the gift to give. She had recently been to Jamaica, visiting a dear relative who was terminally ill, and returned with a cough and shoulder pain from pulling heavy luggage, adding to her arthritis and fibromyalgia (chronic muscle ache). She'd been seen by Dr Newman, who sent her to me to have a steroid shoulder injection.

While I was preparing for the injection, we chatted about her trip to Jamaica, then Mrs Robertson mentioned that she'd received a letter from a central London hospital because she didn't attend her nephrology (kidney disease) appointment. I requested it to her before her trip, but surprisingly there was no appointment letter in the first place.

She rang the hospital to explain that to the secretary, but an automated machine message said, "If you know your extension number, enter it now. If you know the department, say it now." When Mrs Robertson mentioned the nephrology department, the automated voice answered, "Do you mean neurology?" Mrs Robertson replied, "No, nephrology." The machine said, "I'm sorry, please wait for an operator", then the line cut off.

Mrs Robertson told me, "It might be my accent."

I replied, "No, it is not your accent. I used to work for that hospital during my training years ago, and that machine used to do the same thing to me, and I thought, like you, it was my accent. So I asked a colleague, who speaks Queen's English with no accent, and it did the same. The machine can't differentiate between neurology and nephrology, haematology and rheumatology. Probably it has selective deafness, who knows!"

I told her I'd ask our administrators to contact the hospital secretaries about that and gave her the injection.

She gave me a big smile and said, "Thank you" – two simple words worth a lot to us GPs.

* * * * *

I quickly checked my NHS email, and read an invitation to a drug company-sponsored education session in Central London, with a meal afterwards to make sure the doctors stayed to the bitter end, which is very late for me. It made me wonders how on earth doctors can advise patients not to eat late, and then agree to these invitations. Mind you, some doctors smoke – and advise patients not to!

I decided to leave some important emails until the following day. However, I found a message from the local hospital cardiology team about developing a "new pathway". I read it with a cynical, tired brain, as we doctors hear the phrase "improved pathway" many times, along with "upgraded protocols" and "new guidelines", etc., etc.

However, I read all four pages of the "improved pathway" to find at the end of each page a sentence written in bold: **If you have any query contact COD or COW**.

I asked a learned colleague, who was very good at crosswords and abbreviations, what it meant. No idea. So I decided to do something positive with this COD thing, and I texted my wife to order cod and chips for our supper.

I checked the mail for anything that needed to be dealt with before going home, and I found a letter for my attention from our staff. We had referred a lady for a cardiology (heart disease) appointment, but the department returned the referral and requested that the lady have an echocardiogram (heart scan) before seeing a consultant. One of my colleagues then requested the scan, but it was rejected as the patient had to see the consultant first!

With a big sigh, I decided to ring the on-call team to process the scan to avoid any delay – and by the way asking them about COD and COW.

To my surprise, it turned out to be Consultant of Day (COD) or Consultant of Week (COW).

I asked cheekily, "So when I ring for any query, can I ask 'Is he or she the Cod or the Cow?'". The line went quiet.

I hope they got the message!

* * * * *

While I was looking at the screen to call the next patient, I heard somebody shouting and crying, arguing with the reception staff.

I opened the door of my room and the voice was clearer. "I need to see him, he is my doctor!"

The receptionist replied in a calming voice, "He is very busy, you can see somebody else. And please remember, it is not a walk-in service, you have to have an appointment."

I recognised the voice of Rebecca, a hard-working mother of a 13-year-old son. She was a teaching assistant, living a comfortable and quiet life, and came to the surgery sporadically, as she was healthy enough.

I decided to intervene in the dispute between Rebecca and the receptionist, as our practice manager was away. I ushered Rebecca to my room, apologising to my next patient for the delay.

Rebecca sat in the chair, crying, and told me about her partner Colin. He is not one of our patients, and I've never met him, but Rebecca had mentioned him before.

"I'm sorry, I didn't know what to do, and the surgery is the nearest help. I went to work after a weird weekend in which Colin, who was isolating himself in the bedroom, didn't want to go out with his mates, as he usually does on weekends when we don't have commitments. He didn't take our son to a football match in the park, like he usually does. When he was eating with us he hardly talked and seemed far away. Every time I asked him what was wrong, he shook his head and said, "Nothing's wrong". We had trivial arguments a few weeks ago, like any family.

Rebecca added, "I went to the school and left Colin at home, as he was made redundant a month ago from the company where he worked for 12 years. I came home to find he'd collected his belongings and left a note in the kitchen, saying he was walking away from all of it, didn't want to know us anymore, and asking us not to try to find him, and to forget about our 18 years together."

She paused, sobbed, and continued, "I couldn't believe it. I can't find a reason for it. Sorry, doctor, to take up your time."

I consoled her and asked about her son. She replied, "He is with his friend till evening, when I'll collect him."

I asked Rebecca if she had a friend or family to confide in, and she answered, "Unfortunately not. I have a work friend, but not really a close friend, and Mum and Dad are on holiday in Spain. My brother in Wales is busy with his wife and a disabled kid and their responsibilities, and has no time for anything else."

I offered Rebecca an urgent appointment with the counselling service and because she repeatedly said "How am I going to sleep tonight?" I offered her some sleeping tablets and a week off work at the school to try to cope with this shock in her life. I told her to come back after a week if she still needed our support.

* * * * *

My last patient was Angela Copperfield, who was struggling with sleepless nights. My tired brain said, "You're not the only one, Angela."

I hadn't seen Angela for years. She had worked for the Ministry of Defence and didn't like it and its office politics, and decided to change her job. Angela was very well spoken, in her late 40s, and happily married to Steve, an accountant and one of our patients, with two lovely children.

Angela looked very anxious and told me, "I haven't slept well for about a week. I've tried over-the-counter and herbal remedies, meditation and calming music, with little effect. I feel tired but I toss and turn in bed, and I have to get up for the kids and to go to work. I have no appetite for breakfast, and I get headaches every day. I feel my pulse racing, my heart pounding, and I worry that something catastrophic will happen."

I asked what she thought was causing her anxiety.

"Two weeks ago it came to my attention that my daughter had been bullied at school. It made her unhappy and she started fighting with her brother about little things, which makes the atmosphere at home not pleasant. I met the head teacher and things hopefully should settle down soon," she said.

Angela added that her shower floor was leaking badly into the kitchen downstairs and Steve had to ring a builder relative to help. The floor and the whole shower had to be refurbished, turning the house into a building site. Steve was under pressure at work, and his beloved mum had been diagnosed with ovarian cancer four weeks earlier and had started chemotherapy.

"Steve is coping with these problems by drinking too much. He promised to cut down. At least he sleeps at the end, and I'm not."

Angela continued, "It is the stress at my work which is pushing me into a very dark tunnel, where I can't see any light at the end of it. We are short of staff as my deputy has gone on maternity leave, there are many fast-paced changes, and some new software is causing a lot of problems.

"I can't access my emails for the last three days. Despite multiple complaints about the problem, nobody is listening. With deadlines approaching, meetings had to be cascaded and there's pressure from the company headquarters to sort things out.

"Despite repeated complaints that the emails are not working, they reassured us that the engineers were working on the problems but it will take time. Nobody knows when it will be sorted out."

It all sounded very familiar to me.

I suggested that Angela should meet the top managers to explain the situation, and she said she'd already requested an urgent meeting with them.

I said she needed counselling support for her short period of stress and anxiety, which she agreed. She had requested a private one on the company's insurance.

I also prescribed sedating antihistamine tablets, which are not addictive, to help her sleep.

Angela said she was now starting to feel supported and positive, and ready to face the work stress.

I thought 'which company would leave their staff working under these awful circumstances?', and asked her where she now worked.

Angela looked at the floor and said in a weak voice, "I'm the chief IT communications manager of that reputable company which is subcontracted to the NHS."

We looked at each other, eye to eye, in silence, with only the sound of raindrops on the window.

I said, "Let me know if you need more help, Angela. God help us, and good luck."

As she left the room, I thought, "Top communications manager can't communicate through her own email. That says it all."

* * * * *

I stayed on for a few minutes to release the emotion from Angela's consultation, looking at a few letters from the hospital that had been left on my desk.

I noticed that some letters were addressed to Dr Unknown, or Dr Locum or Dr Pooled list, showing the pressure on the system, with some staff having no time to check the name of the doctor they were sending the referral to.

One letter was addressed to Dr Smith, a great colleague who had passed away seven years earlier. We'd mentioned his death to the local and other hospitals repeatedly – but they still sent letters to him!

I suddenly felt hungry and realised that I'd had no break, or even a cup of tea, for a long time. I felt so tired and decided to go home and rest from that heavy rainy day. By the way, that was only three-quarter's of a day's work, as I was cutting down my work hours.

Many of my hard-working colleagues all over the country work until 6:30 or 7pm, and sometimes beyond that. One colleague admitted that he stays after all the staff at the clinic have left, continuing until the cleaner comes into his room.

If the decision makers and top politicians could spend just one day in the surgery, it would certainly help them to understand the many problems of our beloved but ailing NHS.

Thankfully I managed to escape past reception, with last-minute jobs that would definitely wait until the following day, and ran like a rocket to my car. The strong winds of the day had blown dust from the roofs of the surrounding buildings and, with the rain; I couldn't recognised my Jaguar, as it had changed into a spotty leopard.

I reversed the car slowly and I could see in the rear-view mirror the familiar face of a patient, Mr Saunders, with his slow pace and walking stick, with his wife carrying an umbrella for both of them.

Mr Saunders came close to the driver's side to say hello to me, and I wound down the window.

With a wide smile he said, "Thanks, Doc. I got my disability badge this morning.

I replied, "You are welcome." Thank God, a happy costumer, with some good news.

As I drove home, the rain began to fade away, and I was happy to say goodbye to a tense, hectic day, with its constant downpours and swirling winds.

As the 1980s hit pop song said, it was "Just another manic Monday."

However, it had taught me an important thing in life: To raise my words, not my voice, as it is the rain that grows flowers, not the thunder.

* * * * *

John Marshall (part two) – an uplifting story

John Marshall, the gloomy patient with the personal hygiene problem, returned to the surgery after two weeks, and this time I had an ample time for him and his letters, reports, complaints etc.

I noticed John was more positive than the last time, and chatty as well. He passed me the forms for the lower water charges that he'd mentioned the last visit.

While I was going through the forms, John kept on saying that he'd read some parts of them but couldn't understand a lot.

"Am I dyslexic, Doc.?" he asked. "Because if I'm, then the disability people should know and the Job Centre should stop hassling me.

"I remember I hated books at the school. You know, Doc., I even get anxiety from the word book. Last week, after I had few drinks with my mates in the pub, I strolled with one of them; his name is Daniel, my best friend. I've known him for years; he used to work for a computer company before it went bankrupt, or what they used to call it, the bubble burst.

"Daniel invited me for more drinks in his flat on the estate where he lives, which he repeatedly said he hated. It was obvious when he entered the estate and started shouting, 'I'm the greatest, I'm the lion king, I'm the king of the jungle, I'm the king prawn in the ocean, you idiots!' He was drunk, and the people in the estate shouted back at him from their windows, 'Shut up, shut the f*** up!'

"Anyway, while we were drinking in his flat, he was playing with his computer. I was curious and asked him 'Who are these people on the screen?' He explained that it was called Facebook. I said, 'face what?' and he said 'Facebook'. I said, 'Not for me, mate. I stopped dealing with any book since I left school.'

"Daniel patiently explained to me how computers can help us in life. I was sceptical but willing to learn from him. I noticed that he sold a few items on the internet and he asked me sarcastically if I had any items to sell that I didn't need. I joked that I only had my clothes."

I explained the forms to John and signed them for him, hinting that reception might ask him for small administrative fee (non-NHS contract work). John swiftly pleaded having no money, but promised if he did get some soon he'd come back and pay. I was in a charitable mood and allowed him to do so, knowing that some surgeries wouldn't allow this unless the patient pays, and sometimes in advance.

After the session, I thought about his question "Am I dyslexic?" so I went back to his medical record and all I found was that he'd had behavioural issues at school, with repeated fights, detentions and exclusion until he left to work for a big DIY store. There was an entry in his record when he came accompanied by his girlfriend Dawn, as he had been drunk over the weekend and had a fight with some lads in the pub, causing him multiple facial cuts and bruises.

However, there was no reference to learning difficulties or specifically dyslexia, so I asked Veronica, our administrator, to investigate where we could send adult cases for diagnosis, having had difficulties in the past with similar cases. The system kept changing the centre responsible for this diagnosis.

Veronica came back later and said that adult dyslexia fell into a gap in the system, as every organisation she'd contacted would ask her to ask somewhere else. Some tested people until the age of 25 but after that age no funds were available. Some advised her to check with the Job Centre, where an Occupational Health Adviser should be able to help. Veronica tried them, with no luck as they advised her to contact charity organisations, or the patient could go privately, which cost a lot of money, and poor John couldn't afford it.

Veronica said, "The majority of people I asked pointed me towards the websites of voluntary organisations, which had the same information, but the last resource mentioned was www.gov.uk."

When she said the word 'gov' I had doubts instantly, but I decided to be positive and give it a go. With Veronica watching the screen, I typed the web page and up came the page with lots of services, advice and contacts.

We typed 'dyslexia and learning disability diagnosis', and mainly got information about claiming benefits. We needed to talk to someone about which department could help with diagnosis. Eventually there were phone numbers, which made us optimistic. The first number we rang was a dead number! We tried again, same result. The second number kept ringing but nobody answered, and the last number was a recorded message, giving loads of instructions, eventually asking us to contact the local Job Centre for advice!

We noticed that at the end of the page they had the audacity to ask us for feedback about the service.

I asked Veronica, "What service are they talking about? We are back to square one, back to the Job Centre."

* * * * *

A month later, during an administrative session, I noticed John Marshall's name on my list. I called him in and with a broad smile he said, "I got you the money, Doc."

"What money?" I asked.

"The money, for the form filling at my last visit."

I'd forgotten all about it, probably from the increasing pressure of work and mountain of forms and letters on a daily basis. "Thank you, John. You can give it to the reception."

John explained how he now had this surplus of money.

"My friend Daniel visited my flat and found that I had a valuable collection of miniature cars and model trains that I used to collect from car boot sales years and years ago, when I was with my girlfriend Dawn.

"Daniel decided to put a few of them on the internet for sale, and to my surprise many people wanted them, and we got money for them. I gave Daniel some and kept the rest. We repeated this fun, which was better than gambling and equally exciting.

"Then we came up with an idea that I should go to car boot sales and collect interesting toy models, and Daniel would sell them on the internet. We are businessmen now!"

Every time I saw John, I asked him about himself and the internet project, and I noticed he was less smelly, paid attention to his clothes, with some new and some second-hand from charity shops. He was mentally stimulated as he visited more and more car boot sales and charity shops all over London.

I was very pleased with his progress and one day I received a request for a character reference for him, as he'd agreed to do a few hours' unpaid work in one of the charity shops he visited. Having a chat with their staff, I was happy to supply the reference, despite our increasing workload.

John disappeared for a while and then returned for a private letter referral to a learning disabilities consultant to diagnose his dyslexia. As I wrote him the letter, John told me his internet business with Daniel was doing very well, and they dedicated their weekends to car boot sales, getting up early. It kept them busy and their alcohol consumption had been reduced dramatically, and was confined only to business chats in the pub.

I was so happy to see the transformation in John's lifestyle, as he talked about his business rather than his drinking, smoking and gambling.

John paused for a few seconds, as if hesitant to mention something, then continued, "You wouldn't believe it, Doc. One day I decided to write Dawn's name, my ex-girlfriend, in the search field on Facebook, which Daniel taught me, and I was surprised to see her picture. I visited her page and sailed away in a sea of memories.

"The next day I told Daniel about my discovery, and Daniel encouraged me to write a small message to Dawn. I was reluctant, with a fear of rejection, but I wrote, 'How are you?' I waited in anticipation for two days, with no response, until on the third day I received a short message from her, saying 'Hello stranger! Is that you? Apologies for the delay in replying but I was busy in the hospital with Nancy, my seven-year-old daughter, who had her tonsils out'."

A month later, John came back to the surgery with right shoulder pain, from carrying heavy goods at car boot sales. I gave him pain relief and taught him physiotherapy exercises. He was in a very happy mood and mentioned that Dawn was coming to visit some relatives in London and they'd agreed to meet for afternoon tea.

Later on, John, reported on that afternoon tea with mixed emotions, as he'd noticed the effect of the years upon them both, with some changes of their personality and attitude.

Life had taught Dawn to be wise after she had a terrible time with a violent husband, until she got a divorce. She had a daughter, Nancy, living with her.

John and Dawn talked and joked, just like they used to, and he apologised profusely about the final incident in their relationship. He had drunk heavily and fallen asleep on the sofa in the living room, woken up still a bit drunk with a hangover, tried to have breakfast, couldn't find any milk in the fridge so drank white wine instead, watched TV and fell asleep again. For Dawn, it was the final straw.

However, they laughed about it and John admitted he was not that selfish and chaotic person any more, and they agreed to keep in touch regularly.

John said they now talked regularly by Skype and their relationship had grown stronger. They'd agreed that John would visit her and daughter Nancy in Leeds regularly and spend more time and weekends with them.

John transferred his work to Leeds, bought a small old car and rented a small shop, selling old toys and model cars with Dawn's help. They were very settled and living together as a couple.

John wrote a thank-you card to our staff, telling them what he was doing, and then a Christmas card with more good news about his flourishing business, his new baby boy with Dawn, who they'd named Daniel after John's friend.

Daniel was still in touch with them, and he represented their Leeds business in London.

The Christmas card had been hand-made on a computer, with a picture of John, Dawn, Daniel, Nancy and junior Daniel, all dancing in the rain and wind of the North.

John had written a philosophical statement on the card: "Life taught us not only to wait for the storm to pass, but also to dance in the rain."

I smiled at his words. How right he was.

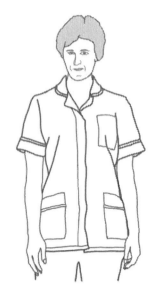

SISTER O'SHEA

Chapter 3

During our medical training we used to move from team to team and from one hospital to another, with each place offering a different mode of work and atmosphere. We soon became acclimatised to the new environments, places and people we worked with.

I started a new job in a university hospital in Birmingham and from the first day after the induction and allocation of every doctor to their places, I tried to collect a few tips from the consultants in the department and the nursing staff. I spoke to many nurses when the time allowed me to – just friendly chats about the weather outside the hospital, then subtly about the atmosphere inside the hospital. I noticed that the name 'Sister O'Shea' was mentioned on many occasions, probably more than the consultants and other staff, and her signature was on many of the written instructions to the nursing staff, on the noticeboard in their sitting room and the nursing station.

I gathered that she got her own way and I did observe the discipline and co-ordination in the ward – you could say that things were run with military precision.

Some time later, I met Sister O'Shea while she was doing the round with the senior consultant and the rest of the team, including the most junior member – me. I introduced myself to her and we all started the round. You could feel the harmony in the ranks and levels of communication between Sister O'Shea and the senior consultant, Dr Mahoney. The round went smoothly, with instructions cascading from the top ranks to the lower ranks, and afterwards I had a brief chat with Sister O'Shea. She asked me the routine friendly questions like "how was your last job?" and "how are you settling in?"

I hinted about her lovely distinct Irish accent, as it reminded me of my time working in Dublin. By coincidence, Sister O'Shea happened to be from there, which put a smile on her face and probably gave me a few brownie points, which I wasn't desperate for, however it was a great bonus.

At mid-day I thought I would be able to sneak off to the canteen for a quick bite and back quickly to finish the remaining work of the morning round. But I was caught by Sister O'Shea, who reminded me about an educational meeting in the lecture theatre. When I told her I would get a sandwich from the canteen and then join the meeting afterwards, she smiled and said, "Lunch is provided and it is free, if you believe in a free lunch! It is supplied by the tycoon drug companies, whose medications you prescribe every day."

That was good news to me, so I finished a few urgent things for some patients and made my way with my colleagues to the lecture theatre, where there were trays of different types of sandwiches, drinks, and brightly coloured posters of the drug company's medications. The drug representative greeted us with a smile, in an effort to catch our attention to talk briefly about their newest medications. I quickly grabbed a few sandwiches and a banana and took my place with the rest of my colleagues.

The lectures went well and swiftly, one after another, sometimes followed by brief questions or a discussion. The last lecture was about memory problems in old age, and at the end the doctor who was presenting it pointed out the increased rate of non-attendance of appointments, where patients were not ringing in advance to cancel. When the doctor asked the managers if they could do something about it, the theatre went very quiet.

Then suddenly a familiar, authoritarian voice commented, "From what I gather, and from an elderly neighbour of mine, who lives alone with the help of carers from the social services, the reason she missed many appointments was actually due to her poor memory. Maybe we could write to their next-of-kin, copying them in on the appointment, just in case the patient who has a poor memory forgot all about it."

I couldn't resist looking at Sister O'Shea, with a broad smile, and she noticed my admiration for her idea. At the end, when we were walking back to the ward, I told her, "You know what? My brain was just thinking that they may appoint an adviser to remind the managers, who in turn will remind the administrators to send a letter reminding the patient with poor memory to remember to turn up to their appointment. But my brain rejected the thought and I was glad to hear your constructive suggestion." Then I joked with her, saying, "What a great idea that was. If we had a few more Sister O' Sheas in the NHS we would be much stronger."

She smiled and accepted the compliment and again I managed to gain a few more brownie points.

The next day I was on call and during the evening round I decided to stay in the ward to finish some new admissions and sort out some investigations. I had the chance to observe the night staff doing their dedicated work. They had to write many entries in their records about the condition of the patients and any events before the routine medications round of the evening. This was to ensure that any additional medications – such as extra painkillers, sleeping tablets or laxatives – could be added if needed. Eventually the ward would go quiet, the lights would be dimmed and people would be ready for a (hopefully) quiet night. This wasn't always the case, as on many occasions there would be a handful of patients in need of extra attention of some sort.

During the week I saw Sister O'Shea and after a brief chat I asked her if I could attend the nursing report meeting to learn more about my patients. I was well aware that it was very unusual for doctors to attend these meetings, as it goes against the culture of work in a hospital environment, and that I was probably asking a slightly cheeky question. But surprisingly she agreed, albeit answering with a little hesitation, saying that she would make an exception to the rule this time and allow me to join.

On my next on-call it was a very busy night and I hardly had any sleep. This sleep deprivation put me in a slightly euphoric mood, like the feeling from a legal high –without paying any money for it.

One cup of tea later and it was time for the nursing report meeting. Sister O'Shea appeared fresh and with her usual firm and authoritarian smile. The nurses reported in detail about each patient and the doctors' instructions and I found it to be very eye-opening for me to learn many aspects about my patients from different angles of care.

Sister O'Shea concluded the meeting and asked if there was any other business to address, looking straight at me. So I thanked her and the nursing team for allowing me to attend, and for the valuable information I had gathered about the patients. I then mentioned that I had noticed the hard-working night staff waking some patients who were already deep asleep, so they could give them their sleeping tablets. I didn't understand the rationale behind that, and I looked at Sister O'Shea, who seemed to understand the confusion behind my observation. Suddenly the nurses understood too, and the whole room burst out laughing.

Sister O'Shea said, "Point taken, Doctor. No need, girls, to wake the patient if they are asleep to give them their sleeping tablets."

With everybody laughing, I had no response except, "It seems that laughter is the best medicine, Sister – and it is free on the NHS."

* * * * *

One day during the round of Dr Mahoney, there was an elderly lady patient, in her early 90s, who'd had major surgery and recovered well. However, she had then contracted a chest infection. So Dr Mahoney had agreed to look after her in his medical ward until she would be discharged to go home.

He asked her how she was doing and she answered, "I'm well and ready to go home. As you can see, my daughter brought me two dresses, which are hanging near the bed, but my only problem now is: which one should I wear?"

Dr Mahoney batted this question to Sister O'Shea. With a smile, Sister O'Shea chose the flowery dress with a dark background.

After we moved from her bed, Sister O'Shea whispered in my ear, "I hope that when I'm 90 years old my only problem will be choosing between two dresses."

The hard work on the ward continued until one day I saw the announcement of Dr Mahoney's retirement party, which I attended. It was an event that raised mixed emotions, between the happiness of him being finished with the mission of long years of dedicated work, and the staff being very sad to see him go.

I heard from some of the staff that about five years earlier he had lost his dear wife after a long fight with cancer. I also heard that Sister O'Shea had been a good friend of hers. Dr Mahoney's only son Patrick had graduated from medical school and after a few years of working for the NHS had decided to go and work in New Zealand with some of his colleagues.

After reducing his hospital duties, Dr Mahoney had more time to dedicate to his charitable work with the local church, where Sister O'Shea was an active member and a regular attendee. I felt happy when I saw them talking to each other, as if she was reassuring him he wouldn't be lonely after his retirement.

A few weeks later I was coming to the ward after finishing the morning outpatient clinics and found Sister O'Shea surrounded by smiling and giggling ward staff. Curious, I decided to ask about the occasion and a senior nurse told me that Dr Mahoney had proposed to Sister O'Shea over the weekend, and they were planning to get married when his son Patrick came over from New Zealand.

Later on I attended Sister O'Shea's retirement party. When I mentioned to her that she was still young, she answered, "I can't handle these fast-paced changes and new management styles. Besides, I have other things to do in life, like taking Dr Mahoney to a lovely, relaxing retirement village near the glorious city of Galway, in the west of our beloved Republic of Ireland."

I smiled broadly and wished them all the very best. They certainly left me with some wonderful, lifelong memories. The most prominent one was the procedure of writing to the next of kin of dementia patients. This had been taken up by the hospital at that time and proven to be very effective. That simple but great idea has been adopted by many hospitals since and has become a routine nowadays.

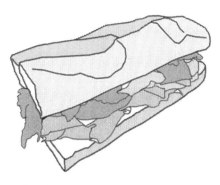

ANY SANDWICH WILL DO

Chapter 4

O ne day I received the monthly newsletter from the writers club of which I'm a member, requesting a piece of writing about food.

Initially I was reluctant to take part, but after a while, with some free time, I remembered something related to food, so I wrote:

In the late 1970s, when I was a medical student, I used to travel around Europe during the summer holidays.

On one occasion I had the chance to work briefly in the vineyards in France to support myself and to help to finance visits to more places. This was where I met a nice young Spanish lady called Rosina. She was married to a French teacher called Didi, who would come for few days at the weekend to lend his wife a helping hand and some moral support with the grape harvest.

We used to have our lunch break together, enjoying the pizza provided courtesy of the vineyard patron. Rosina noticed that I always liked to have the seafood one, and I admitted to her that I was very fond of fish and seafood.

As time went by and the harvest was coming to an end, I told Rosina I would like to visit Spain after I finished working in France. She was delighted to hear of my plans to visit her homeland, and knowing of my passion for all things fishy, she gave me the name of her cousin's fish restaurant in Madrid. She promised to get in touch with him and tell him I would pay him a visit.

I kept the contact details and address, saying I would definitely pass by the restaurant to sample the menu. Then when the work at the vineyard ended and we were all at the farewell party, she told me she had spoken with her cousin and he was looking forward to meeting me. I thanked Rosina and we agreed I would be in Madrid the following Saturday.

I took the train from Marseilles, travelling some seven hours along the coast and finally stopping off at the beautiful city of Barcelona, where I stayed for two days. I had not been there before and spent my time enjoying the amazing art and architecture of the city, the tasty pastries and tapas and the warm and friendly people. Then I caught a train to Madrid, travelling through stunning countryside towards one of the most vibrant cities of Europe and the capital of Spain.

I arrived in the early evening and made my way to the nearest youth hostel, which was apparently not too far from the Plaza del Callao, where Rosina's cousin's fish restaurant was. I signed in, was allocated my bed and had a quick shower before going for a tour of the city to orientate myself. It was a beautiful, warm evening and the city was alive with bright lights, live music and people sitting outside bars and restaurants, enjoying the start of the weekend.

With all the travel and fresh air I slept very well in my humble bunk bed. The next day was Saturday, the day I had arranged to meet Diego, Rosina's cousin. I had a light breakfast at the hostel, not wanting to ruin my appetite for the tasty lunch I was so looking forward to.

I went for a stroll to the tourist information kiosk to get a map of the city. With the help of the friendly information desk staff, I got directions to the Plaza del Callao and the restaurant. They said it was one of the best fish restaurants in the area, and was famous for its speciality menu. Smiling broadly, I tucked the map in my pocket and went to explore the city.

It was another lovely sunny day, not too hot and with a gentle breeze. Ideal for a gentle walk, along many streets, observing the beautiful scenery. There were countless theatres, galleries and museums, beautiful buildings, both historic and modern, shops of every kind and a whole world of restaurants, cafés and snack bars. The vast choice was quite bewildering. But what was definite was that my tummy was reminding me it was time for lunch.

I made my way to the Plaza del Callao and to the little pedestrianised street where the restaurant was. It was very busy, with the usual extension of tables outside, protected from the midday sun by colourful umbrellas. A large smiling fish hanging above the door confirmed I had found the right place.

I went inside and at the bar I saw a tall, handsome man who had the air of a famous conductor, directing his busy staff to meet all his customers' needs. This had to be Diego. As I approached he looked up and rushed towards me, gave me a very warm welcome, and spoke excitedly to me in mixed Spanish and English.

As he led me to a table with a view of the street, he told me that Rosina had spoken very highly of me and said I was a real fish connoisseur. We chatted for a while and he spoke very good English. He explained that he had worked in North London when he was a student, in a fish and chip shop in Kilburn. He had met Maria there, the lady who would later be his wife.

It was very busy in the restaurant and Diego introduced me to a waiter named Alexander, a friendly, smart young man with a pleasant smile and eager attitude. Diego said a few words to him in Spanish and told me he had explained that I was his special guest and should have whatever I wished for.

Alexander brought me a bottle of water and a plate of green and black olives with some fresh bread and butter. He didn't speak any English, but he kept smiling and we managed well with my odd Spanish words I had picked up from Rosina and some sign language.

When he brought me the menu, there was a new challenge for me, as it was written only in Spanish and all my vocabulary was very limited. Mostly I had only two or three words and phrases like "Olla amigo" (hello friend), "mannana" (tomorrow), and that phrase from the song – "Que sera, sera".

But at least I knew it was a fish restaurant and that I liked fish – so all I needed to do was read through the menu until I recognised something. Unfortunately it wasn't quite that simple. Going through the menu line by line I couldn't understand what any of it meant. I was sure it was all delicious but didn't have a clue what to order, and looking around the restaurant I found Diego was nowhere to be seen.

Then I spotted a long sentence, probably describing something special, and alongside it a picture of a fish. Putting the two together I thought this would be the safest choice, so I called Alexander over, pointed at the fish and said, "I would like the fish." Alexander smiled broadly and seemed very pleased with my choice, saying something in Spanish that sounded like 'very good'. He took the menu and dashed off to the kitchen.

I nibbled on the bread and olives, enjoying the scenery in the street, awaiting the culinary treat I had ordered. Alexander soon reappeared at my table, carrying a covered dish which he reverently placed in the centre of the table, as if it was a precious treasure. He nodded at me and said what I assumed meant 'bon appetite' in Spanish, then quickly disappeared, almost like the genie in Aladdin.

I looked at the dish he had presented and at first thought it must be a side dish because it seemed rather small for a main course. But as Alexander did not return, I decided I had better make a start. I lifted the lid to take a look and was met with a cloud of steam with an unbelievably strong smell of fish. As the steam cleared away, all that I could see was a deep bowl of soup with two big fish heads staring back at me. I'm not sure who was more surprised, me or them.

It took a few seconds for me to absorb what was going on. I picked up a menu from a neighbouring table and looked carefully at what I had ordered. The meaning of the words "Sopa de Piscado" suddenly became very clear to me. In my eagerness to find something with fish I had missed the word for soup, assuming that the picture of fish meant just that.

Although I had been hungry, I'd never tried fish soup in my life and was not willing to do so. The overpowering smell and the two fish heads made me lose my appetite completely. I continued nibbling the olives, but pushed the dish to the far side of the table.

When Alexander returned to check on me I tried to explain that I wasn't feeling very well and needed to go. I must have looked pretty rough, as he quickly understood my sign language. When I tried to pay the bill Alexander pushed my hand away, saying "no, Diego, no", clearly meaning his boss had said not to charge. I gratefully accepted the generosity, thanked him and quickly went out to the square for some fresh air.

I found a wooden bench in the shade and watched the crowds of tourists and shoppers. But the sight of the staring fish heads kept coming to my mind and I was convinced I could still smell that pungent soup.

I decided to continue exploring the city to distract myself from the uncomfortable experience. I found myself standing in front of a cinema. It had a big poster on display for a movie called Midnight Express. I had heard people talking about it when I was in France and that it was based on a true story of an American hashish smuggler who escaped from a hellish Turkish jail after being given a 30-year sentence.

I was planning to visit Turkey during the next summer holidays and as I liked true stories I decided to buy a ticket and watch the film. It seemed to be a very popular choice as the ticket booth was very busy, especially as the film was about to start. I bought my ticket, picked up a drink and some popcorn and joined the crowd in the cool darkness of the theatre, leaving my fish soup experience behind me.

At first I enjoyed the film, but soon the story turned dark and very disturbing, with horrific scenes of torture and extreme violence. The crowd repeatedly moaned about the brutality and the very emotionally charged events. By the time the movie finished I had no desire to visit Turkey for many years to come. I left the cinema like a rocket, as if I was escaping from prison myself, with somebody chasing me.

Back in the brightness of day and the fresh air, I felt really hungry – after all, olives, bread and popcorn had not really been much of a lunch, and it was late afternoon. I kept walking until I came to a small supermarket. I went in to pick up anything quick and easy to eat. Near the till was a fridge with many sandwiches and snacks to choose from. I found it hard to decide, but my brain was screaming, "Any sandwich will do – except fish".

I grabbed a cheese and tomato sandwich, paid and left. This did the trick and while I was eating it in the buzzing street I discovered I had learnt something important that day. From now on I would be more careful about reading menus and always say NO to something I didn't like to eat. So I can say to the Spanish "no Sopa de Piscado", to the French "no frogs' legs" and certainly a big no to some of the Far Eastern delicacies of cats or dogs!

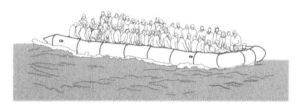

TRIUMPH OVER MANY TRAGEDIES

Chapter 5

I will never forget my first encounter with Fatima Abdullah and her two children: 5½-year-old Mohamed and his four-year-old sister, Aysha. They were recently registered with our practice and had come seeking help, with barely a word of English to communicate their needs. Fatima's friend, who had volunteered to come to translate for her, had disappeared before the appointment, so Fatima came alone.

I greeted her and she answered me with "Salam Alykum" (which means 'Peace upon you 'as a greeting in Islamic religion), followed by "no English".

Realising the immediate problem I reached out for the interpreter phone line on my desk. It was a handy tool that connected with an interpreter who would listen to the patient and then translate to the doctor as if they were in the room. Although it was very helpful I had hardly used it in months, but all I needed was to know which language I needed translating and this was already in her medical record as being Somalian.

With the interpreter on line we started the consultation. Fatima was clearly very distressed, and kept pausing and crying and as I waited to hear her story from the interpreter, all I could do was wait helplessly, provide her with tissues and keep observing little Mohamed, who was looking at me with a shy gaze but with eyes full of fear. Aysha was less fearful and her inquisitive eyes were looking all over the room full of medical equipment.

Eventually the interpreter explained that Fatima couldn't sleep because little Mohamed would keep waking up at night, screaming. Fatima was feeling very sick and couldn't eat. I jumped to question her about her sickness through the interpreter, asking if she might be pregnant.

But when the interpreter conveyed the question, Fatima started to answer and then burst into tears again, explaining to the interpreter that nobody had touched her after the death of her husband. I started to realise that this was a very complex case.

As I listened to the interpreter I concentrated hard and tried to get to the root of the problem and to understand more about the background. Slowly, with many breaks between Fatima's emotional outpourings and the interpreter's translation, the full and harrowing story started to emerge.

* * * * *

Fatima was an asylum seeker, having arrived hidden in a lorry carrying goods to a depot in south-east London. While unloading the cargo with the help of the depot staff, the driver had discovered her and her kids hidden at the back of the lorry between the crates.

The driver and the staff were shocked by the appearance of Fatima and her kids and quickly called the police. They in turn contacted immigration officers and an interpreter arrived, who took all the information needed, and the little family were quickly lodged at a nearby Salvation Army building, together with a few other asylum seekers.

After spending the night there, a lady from social services visited them and advised that they needed to be registered with a GP nearby as soon as possible.

One of the ladies from the group of asylum seekers decided to go with her to the surgery and helped her to fill in the forms and then to book this appointment. But the kind lady had not been able to come with her today.

I decided to give her some sleeping tablets to help her for a few days until she could come back in my administration session to be followed up. I also prescribed sedating antihistamine syrup for Mohamed to help him to sleep at night, hopefully with no nightmares.

Fatima was in her late twenties. She was tall, dark skinned and with attractive facial features, between Middle Eastern and African. Her large deep brown eyes carried a sad gaze and most of the time there was reluctance for eye contact. She wore a head scarf and loose dark brown dress down to her ankles, with only her hands and face exposed and the rest of the body completely covered. On her feet were rough woollen socks with tacky old brown sandals, which were not suitable for the autumn weather of London. Despite her circumstances she carried herself with dignity and there was strength in her.

Later on, when she had been referred for counselling, to help her come to terms with the things she and children had gone through, the bigger picture started to emerge.

* * * * *

Fatima narrated to the counselling staff through an interpreter that in the late 1990s she had been living a quiet life with her husband in a village near the Somali capital of Mogadishu. She looked after the house and the two children, Mohamed and Aysha. They had a large four-bedroom house with a back yard and a big storage barn at the end. Her husband owned some agricultural land and some grazing land for the sheep and goats they had. Things were good for the little family and they lived a peaceful and comfortable life. They had all they needed and were able to give charity to the needy and orphans in the village, over and above that required by the obligatory charity called 'Zakat'. This was an annual amount of 2.5% of the capital a person held and was part of their religious duty.

But times were changing and the quiet life changed slowly as a fear started to go through the village. Soon there were the distant faint sounds of the war, explosions and shooting coming towards the peaceful village. Because of the actions of a few politicians, multiple sects and warlords were fighting each other and many ordinary Somali suffered because of this civil war.

One day Fatima and her husband decided to go to the market in the next town to buy few things for the house. They took Mohamed with them but they left Aysha with her auntie. While Fatima and her husband were walking in the market there was suddenly the sound of a big explosion followed by bursts of random shooting from every direction. Everything happened so quickly that they had no chance to run before her husband, who had been walking beside her, was shot in the chest and fell to the ground in a pool of blood in front of her and Mohamed. Fatima was in shock and didn't know what to do: to grab Mohamed and run for their lives, or to stay and nurse her poor bleeding husband, who was fighting for his life.

Later she found it hard to remember what had happened, as it passed very quickly. All she could recall was the dust surrounding the scene from people running in every direction, the blood everywhere, the screams, the tears, and the fear that filled her body with numbness.

Then suddenly, two strong men appeared from nowhere, put her husband on a wooden hand cart and rushed them towards a waiting car on the top of the street. As one man pushed them into the car the other ordered the driver to take them to the town hospital. Unfortunately her husband died shortly after arrival.

Fatima returned home that evening to feed the hungry kids and put them to sleep. There were now many relatives, friends and neighbours, filling the house with an atmosphere of sadness. For Fatima the terrible feelings of loss and grief were now accompanied by constant insomnia, flashbacks and nightmares. A ghost haunted her and Mohamed in their fitful sleep frequently in the weeks and months that followed.

The burial of her husband took place quickly the following morning and Fatima was invited by the elder ladies of the tribe to meet the wise men of the tribe. Hajj Ibrahim was the tribal elder, and the most respected figure of the village. They were all concerned for the safety of Fatima and her children and in the view of the escalation of the violence which was now threatening to involve the village, Fatima and the children were given the option of flee the village and cross the border into Kenya with other people from the village. Hajj Ibrahim would organise everything for them over the next two days.

Fatima had no option but to accept the offer for the sake of her children's safety. Next day, while she was preparing for the difficult journey, Hajj Ibrahim visited her with two of the elder women of the tribe. He told her that he had contacted some people who would organise the trip, and to Fatima's surprise and relief he added that a cousin of her husband had agreed to buy their land. He gave her a few hundred euros, which was the deposit for the land. The money would be a huge help for the little family on their journey.

The cousin was living in Italy and Hajj Ibrahim gave Fatima his contact details in case she needed to reach him.

Fatima thanked Hajj Ibrahim and asked if he would make sure that the goats were distributed among the remaining family, with half of the sheep being given to the cousin as a gift and the other half to be given for charity for hungry and poor people of the village.

Fatima prepared a small backpack with a few clothes for the children, some dried dates, a little bread and some water for the road. Then she sewed a few gold pieces into the lining of her dress to keep them safe for any emergency. They were especially precious to her as they had been a present from her late husband when they went to Makah in Saudi Arabia on Haj together some years ago. Then she took the euros that Hajj Ibrahim had given her and, wrapping them in a handkerchief, tucked them into her bra for safety. Finally she made sure to wear a piece of Quran around her neck to protect herself and her family on the journey.

* * * * *

The next morning, just as the misty dawn was breaking over the village, Fatima quietly said her prayers and went to wake her children from their innocent sleep. They joined other villagers who were also leaving the warzone behind with hope of a better and safer life somewhere else. They were all squeezed into a battered old pickup truck at the edge of the village and anxiously started their journey into the unknown.

In the crush of the truck it was hard to see where they were going. All Fatima knew was that they were driving for many hours over rough roads and desert tracks, through towns and villages she had never seen. At each place more trucks joined them as they formed a ragged convoy heading for the border with Kenya.

It was probably late afternoon when they stopped briefly to refuel at the last town before the border. Everyone climbed out of the truck, desperate for air and trying to buy a little food or water. But there was no time as they were quickly herded back into the vehicle and the truck rumbled on for the last 50 miles to the border.

Here everyone was told to get out and walk the rest of the way and the truck disappeared behind them in a cloud of dust. Bewildered, exhausted and hungry, they joined the endless stream of people, carrying with them what little they still had, crossing from Somalia to Kenya and the relative safety of Dadaab, one of the world's biggest refugee camp.

There were so many tents, as far as the eye could see, with countless people of all ages, flooding in from every direction, being met by aid workers, trying to register them and allocate them a place to stay.

Fatima and her children, desperately hungry and tired from the long rough journey, were so grateful for two small sandwiches of beans and water they had been given to eat until they were settled the next day. Fatima gave the sandwiches to the children and ate a few of dates from her bag with a little bread and finally succumbed to sleep.

She was awoken by the children, tugging at her clothes and telling her that a very tall man was standing outside the tent and asking about her. Blinking in the bright sunlight, Fatima found that he was the driver of a cattle truck, organised by Hajj Ibrahim, to take them for the next part of their long and exhausting journey towards South Sudan, then onwards towards Libyan border.

They would be travelling with a few other people hidden in the back of the truck behind boxes and cases with varied contents for export. Fatima and a few other people would be in the far corner of the truck. Fatima gave the driver some euros as agreed with Hajj Ibrahim and climbed into the truck with her children, trying to find a comfortable space for what would be a very long and rough journey in cramped, hot conditions.

The truck drove for many days and nights, only stopping briefly to refuel. They were told to stay in the truck and keep quiet so nobody would find them and were only allowed out briefly at night when the driver would stop to take a break at the side of the rough road. He warned them not move far from the truck because they could be kidnapped by bandits or attacked by wild animals. The children were terrified and Fatima did her best to comfort and distract them with stories of a new home in Europe. Fatima was worried too, the food was running out and she had no idea how much longer they would be on the road. She had decided to fast during the day for most of the journey, as if it was the month of Ramadan (the fasting month for Muslims), giving the priority for food to the children.

Eventually they arrived at a deserted village where they were taken from the truck to a van which was dark, cramped and smelly. They could hear that there was some kind of argument between the two drivers and then the van driver opened the door and asked for more money to continue the journey. They tried to explain they had already paid, but he threatened to throw them out of the van and leave them in the road. So they had no choice but to pay.

Once again they were on the road for the long drive to Libya, only interrupted by brief stops on the road, until they reached the Libyan border.

* * * * *

They entered Libya by night, and under the cover of darkness made their way north to the coast and the final destination of an abandoned farm at the edge of an unknown town. The doors of the van were opened and the ragged bunch of weary travellers was hustled out into the bright morning light. Fatima could see many people coming to surround the van and at first she thought they were the workers of the farm. But soon she realised that they too were refugees, all awaiting their turn to cross the sea, which sparkled in the distance.

Fatima and the children stayed there for two days until the boat that would carry them was ready. The traffickers demanded a lot of money in advance and left her with only a hundred euros to continue her journey. Finally, at mid-night, a man came in a pickup truck and took them with about a dozen of the refugees towards the seashore, where a rubber boat that already seemed to be full of refugees was waiting. Despite the boat being already heavily loaded with passengers they were pushed aboard and squeezed in at the very edge. Fatima's whole body felt numb with fear, neither she nor the children could swim and she had no idea how far the boat would need to go across the inky black waters.

Slowly the boat left the shore with its small motor roaring in protest at the heavy load. The huddled passengers all looked frightened and apprehensive, but silently accepted their fate. Mohamed and Aysha clung onto their mother's dress as the lights on the shore grew fainter and eventually disappeared from view.

After a long while they had all got used to the drone of the engine and some had fallen into a fitful sleep out of sheer exhaustion. So when suddenly the engine died and the boat drifted to a stop, the silence was deafening and everyone was instantly awake and alert.

They were motionless on the gently rising and falling waves for what seemed like many hours. Some of the people were moaning with sea sickness and others were mumbling fearful prayers. A breeze was picking up now and the waves were increasing and everyone could feel the fear and panic rising on the little boat in the vast sea.

Fatima hugged her children close and felt them shivering in the bitter cold. It was all she could do to comfort them, hiding her own fear with gentle prayers for God to keep them safe. She had heard the stories of boats like theirs becoming stranded when the fuel ran out and capsizing in the rough seas, with everybody drowned. Closing her eyes to shut out the terror she tried to remember how as a child she used to love being near rivers, the sea and any water, but now that sea was like a huge beast awaiting to swallow them all up at any time it wanted. It was a horrible feeling with every roaring wave, and all that she could do was to continue mentioning Allah and asking him to protect them from any danger.

Fatima wasn't sure if she had dozed briefly with the utter exhaustion, but suddenly became aware of a new sound above the wind and waves, the steady beat of the rotors of a helicopter coming towards them. As she looked up she saw its searchlight cutting through the darkness and heard somebody talking over a loudspeaker. She could not understand what was said as it was in a language she didn't know, but as suddenly as it had appeared it disappeared back into the darkness, leaving only the sound of the sea.

After some time somebody noticed the lights of a ship coming towards them at speed. Some of the passengers started to shout and wave, thinking it would run them down and capsize their overloaded boat. But as it slowed down a searchlight was turned on them, and the boat drew alongside them. There were people in uniforms aboard, again speaking a language Fatima could not understand. Fatima was so afraid, she had heard of pirates ambushing small boats. She felt suddenly very sick and turned her face towards the sea and vomited.

Everything started happening very quickly then. The combination of fear, extreme cold and exhaustion made Fatima feel confused and faint. All she could think about was clinging on to her two children to keep them safe. As she hugged them close she could feel their little bodies shivering and whispered reassuring words in their ears.

The ship was an Italian coastguard vessel sent to pick up the refugees. The crew dropped ladders down to them to climb up, but many were too weak to do so. Those who could stand up carefully, trying not to tip the boat and helped others climb up to the ship. One by one each of them made it to the deck of ship. When her turn came Fatima was at first reluctant to let go of the children, but the kind face of a uniformed lady, reaching down to help, reassured her. Soon they too were sitting on the deck, wrapped in blankets handed out by the crew.

There were nurses on the ship too, checking the refugees for injuries and taking aside those who needed treatment. Fatima was unsure why she was being led away from the group and only realised later that she was bleeding heavily. At first she was confused, not remembering having been injured in any way, but then noticed it came from her underwear and trousers. It seemed she had had a heavy period with clots, but once the nurse had examined her in private and given her clean clothes and some sanitary pads, she explained (through an interpreter on board) that Fatima had had a miscarriage. This was a terrible shock and blow to Fatima, as she had had no idea she was pregnant, and the loss, added to all the other tragic events, would affect her deeply throughout the rest of her life. But for now she would have no time to mourn this little lost soul.

When the ship reached land Fatima and the children were taken to a refugee reception building, where they were quickly registered and provided with food, drinks and beds to sleep. In the morning more detailed information was taken from them and the slow asylum process started.

* * * * *

While waiting to have their paperwork completed, Fatima started to look for a way to contact her husband's cousin. She eventually heard from some of the other refugees that he was living in the north of Italy, but had sent a message for her to sit tight and wait for him to organize her next move. The plan was for her to travel on to France and from there to go to England because the opportunities for her and children would be better there, with access to social benefits, free health care and free education for the kids.

The cousin arrived one weekend and explained the plan to her, giving her some pocket money for the journey. He took them over to a battered old white van and told her that the driver, a large, rough looking man, had been paid and would drive them to France. He warned Fatima that if they were stopped by the police the driver would deny all knowledge and say he didn't know them and she would need to say she didn't know him either. Certainly she couldn't say that he had been paid to take them to France .He would deny everything and say that he had left his van unattended and they had probably got into it. If all was well he would take them all the way to a city called Calais, on the coast. Here it would be up to them to try to cross to England.

The cousin paid the agreed money to the driver and Fatima and the children were once again on the road, huddled in a dark vehicle, not knowing what would happen next.

They travelled for many long hours. The driver made very few stops for them to take some air, relieve themselves or find something to eat or drink. Finally, exhausted and disorientated, they were dumped in the middle of the night on the outskirts of an unfamiliar town, in another foreign land. The driver waved vaguely in the direction of what appeared to be a rough campsite and hastily drove away, leaving the little family to make their own way.

The children were tired and frightened and very hungry and Fatima decided to walk towards the town to find somewhere to buy some food. She managed to find a small shop still open and was just able to afford some bread and some cheese and a bottle of water, which she gave to the children. They sat on a wooden bench and Fatima tried to figure out what she needed to do next. She had almost no money left and did not speak the language. She did not know anybody who might help and suddenly felt very alone in the world. It was the first time that she really felt that she regretted leaving her home and starting this journey into the unknown. But then she felt the piece of Quran around her neck, and looking down at the children drifting off to sleep she knew she had to trust Allah and continue for them. She covered their little bodies with her dress and despite her own tiredness watched over them all night.

As dawn broke she quietly said her prayers and for the first time looked around to properly see where they were. She spotted an African-looking young man, thin and scruffy with dirty, torn clothes and broken shoes held together with string. He was rummaging through the dustbins at the side of a pizza shop, probably looking for any discarded food. Despite his appearance, he seemed quite peaceful and when he noticed her watching a broad smile crossed his face. He disappeared briefly behind the bins and then reappeared with a small plastic bag and crossed the road towards them.

For some reason Fatima did not feel afraid and waited for him to approach. Again he smiled and opened his bag to reveal a mixture of food scraps he had managed to scavenge and offered them to Fatima. The children had woken and were squinting in the early sunlight. Fatima accepted his generosity humbly and they all ate the little breakfast together.

She thought at first he might also be from Somalia, but although he seemed to understand some of her words, he replied in a different language. So she tried a few words of Arabic she had learned from the Quran and a visit to Saudi Arabia many years ago. Adding some sign language and gestures they managed to communicate enough for the young man to find out he was called Ahmed and had come from the Tigray region of Ethiopia, on the border with Eritrea.

Ahmed was only in his mid-teens and had arrived at the camp a few months earlier with a few refugees from his village. The war between Eritrea and Ethiopia had been very violent and resulted in disease and deep poverty throughout the area. When his mum died when their small home was burned down, he fled to Sudan with his dad and started the same perilous journey that Fatima has made.

Sadly his father drowned when their boat capsized in rough seas. Ahmed made the rest of the journey alone, heading for France as he wanted to join his uncle in Manchester in England.

Ahmed had been traumatised by the tragic deaths of his parents, and had struggled to eat and sleep due to his nightmares and flashbacks. It was only because of the very kindness of people he met during the journey that he had had the energy to continue and make it this far alone. Now his only dream was to make it to England and be reunited with his uncle, his only remaining family. It was literally the light at the end of the tunnel; the tunnel that led under the sea to the UK.

Ahmed understood the struggles Fatima had faced to get this far and decided he would try to help them. He helped her carry her small bundle of belongings and took them to the straggling city of tents on the edge of the town where a diverse community of refugees had gathered waiting and hoping for their chance to walk through the tunnel or to hide in the back of any of the lorries heading for England. As Fatima walked slowly behind Ahmed, holding tightly to the hands of her children, she could feel the desperation and fear in the air. It was a feeling that had followed them throughout the journey, but here there did seem to be some light of hope.

Ahmed introduced Fatima to some of the people in the camp who he had become friends with and who welcomed her and her little family to join them. They found them a bit of space in a recently vacated tent, telling her that the boys who had occupied it had only left for England that last night. In a neighbouring tent an elderly man saw the kids and kindly gave them some wrinkly skinned tomatoes and couple of shrunken cucumbers. Later on Fatima learned that he would search for them in the fields the neighbouring farms at night, where imperfect crops were discarded by the workers during the day.

Fatima also heard a lot of horror stories of rape, sexual exploitation, sex trafficking, violence and death, but she closed these from her mind, trusting in her strong belief that she was protected by the Quran around her neck and her faith in Allah. Fatima was determined to be positive for the sake of her children and constantly held the dream of a better future for all of them in her heart and mind.

* * * * *

The little family grew used to the camp and settled into a routine of searching for food and supplies for daily survival and keeping a watch for news of chances to leave. To occupy her mind and repay the many kindnesses she had received, Fatima decided to share a bit in helping others even less fortunate. So she would take the kids walking towards the city centre around lunch time to pass by the various restaurants and shops to check their bins for whatever edible scraps she could bring back for the kids and others in the camp. Sometimes she would see that there would be charitable workers visiting the camp near the main entrance, providing food, drinks, used clothes and blankets. She would then go to receive some for the kids and distribute the rest to others in the camp, especially her neighbour, whose health had worsened in the poor conditions and was no longer able to leave his tent to help himself.

Fatima spent days and weeks in that camping area, hearing mostly about the failed attempts of Ahmed and his young friends who were trying almost every day, day and night. But finally the time came for Fatima to start trying. But it wasn't safe to walk through the tunnel with two small children.

A man in the camp she didn't know advised her to pay any driver some money to take them in his truck and one day he introduced her to an Asian-looking driver of a blue van, who offered to take them to England. Fatima didn't have enough euros to pay what he asked, even when she asked

Ahmed to help her to sell a bracelet of gold she had. He took her to the city shopping area where he managed to find a jewellery shop to buy the bracelet. But the owner realised that there was no proof for ownership so he only agreed to pay a fraction of the price. But Fatima was still a few euros short of her fare and the driver still insisted on the full price. Her neighbour discovered her problem and insisted on her taking some money from him, saying he would not need it as he could not travel and wanted the repay her kindness and see the children safe. Fatima tried to refuse but he insisted and reluctantly she agreed.

In the early dawn the driver came and took the money in advance, despite Fatima and Ahmed's pleas to take the money when they arrived in England. But he insisted on the money in advance, in case the police caught them. So they climbed into the back of the van and hid again behind a pile of packing cases.

After about an hour or so and the van suddenly stopped and the doors opened and Fatima and the children blinked in the sudden light. The driver shouted at them to get off quickly as they had arrived in England. They struggled as he pushed them out, quickly closed the doors and drove off in a cloud of dust and stones. As they looked around them, expecting to see a new land the poor Fatima was horrified to realise that they had been dumped back on the outskirts of the camp. The driver had just driven around for a while, and then dropped them back where they started.

Fatima realised the trick and was shocked that there were such cruel and greedy people who would steal from the desperate, and she started crying helplessly, repeatedly asking why this had happened to her and what religion taught you to take the money of the needy and orphans unfairly. She kept crying all the way back to the camp.

Ahmed learned about this incident and sympathised with Fatima. He promised to help her in any way he could to make sure they made it safely to England. He told all the people in the camp about what had happened to Fatima, whose kindness had touched so many of them, and that they needed their help to take the next available chance to leave.

He came the next day to Fatima and told her the news that the camp was expecting a charity convoy from London. But they were a bit late in arriving. There had been an accident on the road approaching the camp between a lorry and a blue van. The driver of the blue van had unfortunately been badly hurt and transferred by helicopter to the nearest hospital. Thankfully the lorry driver had been ok. Fatima's eyes opened wide in shock and felt very bad and guilty for thinking so badly of the man who conned her and could be the driver of the same blue van. However, she was relieved to know that the driver had been taken to hospital.

When the charity convoy finally arrived Fatima noticed it was being run by a large group of mostly Asian people, smiling and giving away new and old clothes, sleeping bags and plenty of food. She thought deeply and reminded herself that good people and less good people can come from the race or country or continent, just like the disaster at home where brothers, fathers and sons were even fighting and killing each other now. She humbly accepted the food and some clothes, and then noticed that the charitable people also gave her and the children some money, which compensated her loss of what she paid the Asian driver. She made a silent prayer to forgive the driver and ask forgiveness for her own thoughts.

Following the incident with the driver of the blue van, Fatima and children did not have enough money to find someone else to help them. There was no way for a woman alone to make any more money except by immoral means that Fatima would never consider. She would have to find another way. Ahmed and his friends were young and brave enough to attempt the tunnel route, but Fatima and the children could not risk it. Eventually it was decided they would have to risk trying to smuggle themselves onto one of the goods lorries waiting at the port. This was not easy, due the fences and security surrounding the waiting area, and the drivers were very careful because of the trouble they could get in for being negligent in guarding their trucks. It had to be done under cover of darkness, trying to avoid the patrols with their dogs. Ahmed and his friends kept a watch for a suitable chance. It meant that Fatima had to be ready every night to move quickly and had moved her tent closer to the perimeter.

* * * * *

One moonless night Ahmed came to her and said they had to go, now. He led her though a hole in the fence to a small truck. The doors at the back were slightly open and two of Ahmed's friends were waiting. The driver had gone to use the toilets at the other end of the waiting area and the men had broken the lock. They quickly lifted Fatima and the children into the back and told her to hide. The doors closed and they were left in complete darkness. Fatima heard the friends run away and someone shouting at them. Someone rattled the doors but they seemed to be locked. Fatima's heart was beating like it was about to burst from her chest, she was frightened. She covered the children with her dress pushed herself down over them behind the cargo, praying silently for their safety.

Again they were on the move, the truck stopping sometimes for a long time, and then moving again. Fatima had no idea if it was day or night, nor how long they had been travelling. She just kept hidden and didn't move. Thankfully the motion kept the children sleeping.

Fatima too drifted into a fearful sleep, only waking when she felt the truck stop and the engine fall silent. There were a lot of men talking outside – another language she could not understand. But they sounded agitated and there was the sound of a dog barking excitedly. Fatima froze; she knew this was bad news. The doors of the truck swung slowly open and someone pointed a bright torch into the back of the truck, searching out what had alerted the dog, who was straining to jump up. Fatima was blinded by the light and couldn't see who was holding it. But the voice was gruff and demanding and she understood they had been discovered and were being told to come out.

As Fatima and children stood shivering in the depot yard next to the truck, the police arrived, along with immigration officers and people from social services. Fatima and the children were given blankets and led to a hut where a lady tried to talk to Fatima. Fatima could not understand or say anything, she just held the children closer. Eventually another woman arrived who was able to translate and explain to Fatima that she had arrived in the UK and would need to provide as much information as possible so they could process her asylum application. Fatima just nodded in relief – they had finally made it.

* * * * *

Fatima and the children were eventually placed in a women's shelter run by the Salvation Army, neighbouring our surgery. And that's how she came to be one of our patients.

As time went by, they started to settle down a bit and with the support of the social services team, who were already under huge pressure, the children started to attend school. Fatima, with the help of fellow asylum seekers and acquaintances from the shelter, started to get to know her surroundings and took the kids to school every day, visiting the supermarket to get what she needed, and visiting the local mosque for Friday prayers. Here she met people and told them her story and was given support and encouragement. She started learning a few English words, remembering some of them from her childhood in school in Somalia. She had not continued her studies as she had left school to help in her family's business and to eventually get married.

At first Fatima used to say the few English words she knew with no reference to the past or future, with no sentences or grammar. But she was very determined to be understood and did not give up. She would come to me at the surgery each time with a little more, telling me things like 'me go school', 'me shops', 'me eat tablets', 'me sleep', or 'Mohamed no good, no listen', supplemented with a hand and face gesture and some sign language.

I used to struggle sometimes to understand the meaning and when I repeated slowly back to her what she meant to say she would either agree or try again until both of us would be happy and in agreement. If we really got stuck we would use the phone interpreter to translate. However, Fatima was reluctant to do this and as time went on I could see her using more words and sentences and fewer hand and face animations, so I would encourage her and nod, reassuring her that I understood what she meant.

I have to admit that seeing Fatima's progress gave me great inspiration, as if seeing a strong and very determined seed planted in a hostile soil and bad conditions. It was clear that the seed was not only surviving but growing into a strong tree with healthy fruit. What an achievement.

* * * * *

Fatima and the kids were eventually allocated a flat by the council, and according to Fatima's description it was an old one with some damp patches and mould around the windows. There was some damage to the walls and doors, but Fatima wasn't complaining. To her it was all she had wanted; a place that was 'safe'. She said that when she closed the door she knew that they could sleep with no gunshots or explosions, no screams of wounded and dying people, no fear of attack. It was only the occasional nightmares that Mohamed still had in his sleep, running to sleep with her for comfort, which took her back to the past misery.

Fatima used to bring Helen, her neighbour, to translate for her sometimes when Fatima had complicated things to explain. Then when Fatima started talking more for herself she came less frequently. I witnessed the improvement in Fatima, mixed with her struggle to adapt to a different culture and way of life. It seemed harder for her to adapt than for her children. They were doing well at school and had quickly mastered the language.

As time went by she no longer wanted an interpreter, insisting on explaining things herself, eager to practice what she was learning and her growing vocabulary. I was happy to accept the risk of misunderstanding as long as I documented everything in her notes. It was after all 'patient choice' that mattered, and I just did my best to ensure that nothing could go grossly wrong.

There were still occasions, however, when there could be some little misunderstanding.

In subsequent consultations, despite my observation of her huge improvement in English, I discovered there could still be some challenges. One day she mentioned that she had a 'high fever in the nose', only for me to discover that she meant she had 'hay fever of the nose', something she had only developed since she came to London. I guessed that it might be down to different pollens and trees to those found in Somalia.

Another day she came to ask for her asthma 'inhalator', meaning inhaler. Then she had a scan and mentioned that she had been told she had a 'small fibre'. This made me confused for a second as to what kind of fibre she was talking about. Seeing my puzzled face she thankfully pointed towards her lower tummy and I realised she meant 'fibroid', which I confirmed from her record.

On another occasion she mentioned she had been in the bank and had got 'pain in the bonus'. My brain linked bank and bonus and again I got confused. When she pointed to her thighs, the penny finally dropped, she meant 'pain in the bones'.

Around September she came to ask me for a 'flu job' which, after more experience, I quickly realised it was the flu jab she was referring to. There were many other examples, which sometimes made us both laugh; a word with similar pronunciation but different meaning like buy and boy or hair and her. But her good humour and determination helped her to overcome the language barrier.

A different, more sensitive barrier came when, in the course of a consultation, I needed to examine her body. Due to the requirement of modesty from her faith, she was covered from head to toe and I could not ask her to undress. I told her that we had two very good lady doctors who could examine her, as it was sometimes necessary to see or touch the site of any problem. However she was adamant that she only wanted to see her doctor, Dr Moss. So eventually we agreed to examination through the clothing with the offer of a female chaperone if she felt she needed one. If I felt there could be anything serious I would have to insist that one of the ladies at least did the examination. She understood my concerns and finally agreed.

I was very happy about Fatima's good progress and her fast acclimatisation with the new surroundings. I saw frequently as she was afflicted by many diseases, like hay fever, asthma, vitamin D deficiency and a small uterine fibroid. Early on, the more difficult issues were the post-traumatic stress, anxiety and depression, especially when she was communicating regularly with her late husband's cousin about her family back home. He had informed her about the death of Hajj Ibrahim and the departure of her older sister to Somaliland, where there was no war and it was safer. She worried a lot about them all.

Then Fatima developed chronic, widespread body pain, fatigue and poor sleep. She received a diagnosis of fibromyalgia, a disease marked by chronic muscular pain and tiredness, with no known cause, needing treatment with painkillers and gentle exercise and any other help for additional symptoms. It was a blow to this active lady, but she refused to give in and was still strong for her family and capable of giving some of her time to charity work and helping the people around her.

* * * * *

However, the one I was more worried about was poor Mohamed. When he started going to school he used to cry and cling tightly to his mother's clothing. With all the terrible experiences of his young life he was now struggling with a form of separation anxiety. It took a lot of help from the school staff and encouragement from his classmates before he was able to go in.

When Fatima attended a parents' evening, taking a friend with her to translate, it broke her heart to see many dads around and no dad for Mohamed. She explained to me that it was not allowed to have a partner in the Islamic religion, only a husband. But she felt she was not yet ready to marry again and was dedicated to bringing up her children. It was not uncommon for some women in the Middle East and Africa not to remarry after their husband died, especially when they have children. Then she added that she had heard that some husbands may only marry to have the right to stay in the country, and would abandon their wives as soon as they had that right. This worried her a lot. Usually a woman would be introduced to a suitable and respectable man by her family, but here she was alone.

As time passed Mohamed sadly continued to struggle at school and was often behind the class. Then there was an incident where two boys assaulted him, beating him up in a street near the school when he was on his way home. They ran away, leaving him with scratches and bruises all over his hands and legs, but able to make it home. He was so upset he couldn't stop crying all evening and didn't want to go to school the next day. Fatima tried to comfort him but he pulled away from her and didn't want to talk about it. At home he started to increasingly isolate himself in his room as soon as he came home from school, saying he was doing his homework. He would only come out when it was time to eat and was very quiet, answering questions with one word or a nod, then returning to his room. One day Fatima saw him crying in his room and he told her he hated school. Eventually he told her that for a few months now one boy at school had been bullying him repeatedly. Mohamed was really distressed and kept crying. But when his mum tried to gently talk with him he would stop and again refuse to talk about it.

Mohamed became more and more withdrawn from the outside world. His communication with Fatima became very limited and soon he seemed almost emotionless.

Fatima decided to take a friend to translate and went to the school to tell them about the bullying. Initially the school dealt with the issue, but after many weeks it happened again, but with a different boy who called Mohamed a donkey and coward. Once again Fatima informed the school and they dealt with the matter. But these incidents caused Mohamed a lot of anxiety and resulted in poor self-esteem, which was reflected on his attendance record.

At this point Fatima came to tell me about the repeated absences of Mohamed from school and his poor achievement academically. She was so worried and had not known who to turn to. So I wrote a letter to the school to support him and explain the situation. I also requested that they arrange an appointment with a CAMHS (Child and Adolescent Mental Health Services) representative for him at the school. The assessment was done and he was referred for speech and language therapy. After another lengthy assessment they agreed to a diagnosis of learning difficulties and sadly I wasn't surprised. The school were then given measures to take in order to support Mohamed's education better.

* * * * *

When the children were at school Fatima kept herself busy with her charitable work and made many friends in the community. Her English improved so much she was able to help others less able to speak for themselves and helped them to adjust to their new lives. Her kindness and generosity often outweighed her own worries and struggles.

One day she was due to come for her smear test appointment. It had been worrying her for some time, even though our nurse had explained the procedure was very important for her health and generally quite short and painless. However, Fatima was still very apprehensive about the procedure, so she had asked her neighbour and close friend Helen to accompany her. However, on the day Helen told her she couldn't come and Fatima ended up not attending. It was only later that Helen told her what had happened.

Helen was an Eritrean refugee who had escaped the Eritrean-Ethiopian war. She arrived in the UK a long time before Fatima, escaping the death, torture and rape happening in her country. She had had a very lucky escape when some soldiers had captured four women from her village, including Helen. After they had killed all the remaining men in front of their eyes, they told the women to strip and started raping them one by one. As Helen was awaiting the inhumane and barbaric act which would happen to her, she was crying and holding on the cross of her necklace, praying for help and rescue. Suddenly she heard shooting from many directions and the soldiers ran to find a shelter, leaving the women naked on the side of the street.

Helen instinctively grabbed her clothes and just ran in the opposite direction. Later, traumatised by her experience, she couldn't remember anything, apart from joining a small group of crying and screaming folks at the far edge of the village, all running for their lives. It was the start of another very long, exhausting and extremely dangerous journey to eventually reach the safety of England.

Helen had learned Italian and English at school in Eretria and could read and write English reasonably well. She was the one who helped Fatima to write a letter of apology to me for not coming for her appointment. When Fatima next came to me she explained the strange and very disturbing reason for her missing the appointment.

A few months earlier Fatima had celebrated with Helen and the other refugees that Helen had been granted the status to stay and work legally in the UK, something she waited for patiently for very long time. So now she was able to apply for jobs and was finally accepted by a well-known fast food chain. She passed the training and started working lots of different shifts. It was a zero hours contract, meaning they could contact her any time for any shift, and most were very unsociable and long hours. But Helen was just happy to be able to work and have her own income.

However, the previous week she had been called in at short notice to work one of the late evening shifts, from 7pm to 11pm. When she finished she waited for the bus home at the nearby bus stop. It was cold, drizzly and windy and the bus wasn't coming. So, as it was only two bus stops to her home, rather than stand in the cold rain it might be quicker to walk across the park, which should have taken only about 10 minutes longer than the bus journey.

At this time of night the park was deserted and very dark. The path was only dimly lit by the few working street lights. Helen pulled her coat tighter and walked quickly along the path, focusing on the exit gates she could just about see.

In the middle of the park she was confronted by a man in his mid-forties, dressed in dark clothes and wearing thick glasses. In the dark and rain she hadn't noticed him sitting on the wooden bench, drinking a can of beer. She was shocked when he suddenly jumped in front of Helen, grabbing hold of her arms firmly and hoarsely threatened to kill her if she screamed. She was terrified but tried to resist him and escape, but he was very strong, almost double her size and taller than her. He forcefully pushed her behind a big tree and into some bushes where nobody could see them. It all happened so quickly, but to her horror she knew what would happen next. He violently undressed her and raped her before just walking away, as if nothing had happened.

Helen was so shocked that for a moment she could not move, or think or breathe. Eventually she gathered her remaining strength to dress herself and to walk away from the scene, dragging her legs slowly until she found herself in front of Fatima's door. She barely had the energy left to knock and when Fatima cautiously opened the door due the late hour, she just fell in to Fatima's arms crying uncontrollably.

When she was able to finally tell Fatima what had happened, Fatima advised her not to go back to her flat or to wash. Instead they went together to the nearest police station to report the terrible crime. The police took all information Helen could remember. She described the man as accurately as she could, trying to force herself to remember any detail, despite the anguish it caused her. He was taller than her, very strong and heavily built, wearing a hooded jacket. Although the hood concealed a majority of his features he seemed to be of mixed race. She also remembered his deep, rough voice and overpowering smell of alcohol and cigarette smoke. But there was one thing that she remembered as clear as if it had been day. All through the experience she had seen the bright gold cross around his neck, catching the dim light coming through the tree leaves. It had confused her, how could someone wear a cross and still do such an evil thing. It had seared itself in her memory, bringing back the horrors of her past.

The police did what they needed to do but said that the description she had given did not fit anybody on their sex offender's register in that area. They said they would do their best to help Helen, and would be in touch if they had any more information.

Helen was devastated and didn't go to work any more. She was very depressed and traumatised and fearful of leaving her home. This time it was Fatima who went with her to see her GP to help her get counselling and medication if needed. Helen eventually requested that the council help her to move away from the area because it was now filled with only memories of that night. Fatima never mentioned her again, just saying she had moved to somewhere in the north of England.

* * * * *

Mohamed and Aysha were growing up fast now. Mohamed had passed the SATS exams (Standard Attainment Tests) with difficulty and had been accepted in the state secondary school a mile away from their house. At first things were going reasonably well at the new school, but as time went on and with peer pressure and struggles of the puberty, Mohamed was again showing signs of anxiety. Fatima told me that one day he came home crying and told her that one of the boys had told him in front of everybody that Mohamed was a Muslim and all Muslims were terrorists.

Mohamed didn't answer him, he just felt angry, humiliated and embarrassed in front of his friends. He just turned away and ran home, crying angry tears all the way. He locked himself in his room and Fatima could hear him throwing things and shouting. He refused to eat and didn't want to go to school any more.

Fatima was very sad, crying during the consultation, and said she had gone to the school the next day and told them about the incident and why Mohamed was absent for the day.

She tried to tell them that Islam was a religion of peace, not of killing.

She sat in the office, emotionally explaining that what happened to her family and herself was the result of this misunderstanding and the stupidity of the extremists who claimed that they knew Islam very well. Then why did they forget or deliberately ignore that fact that their prophet Mohamed had instructed Muslims not to kill even one person, even during the war he had instructed his soldiers not to harm a tree, women, children, the elderly and anyone who sheltered in a house of worship. Fatima shook her head saying that these extremists, which could be found in any religion, were not the majority and that belief in a religion didn't mean you were a terrorist.

Fatima started crying again about her son and I tried to sympathise with her, saying that the school understood very well what she was saying to them. But Fatima added that they probably did know but they were not doing anything about it. Mohamed had heard the father of the boy was on the board of school governors and very respected by the school. Fatima shrugged and looked at the floor. I couldn't say anything really but understood what she was saying.

Mohamed's anxiety and anger were getting worse, so I decided to help them and wrote to the school, highlighting the background of the family and requesting input from their school nurse and a referral to CAMHS again.

A few weeks later the school nurse wrote to me to acknowledge the situation, kept the information in the school record and requested that the surgery refer Mohamed to CAMHS.

So I made the referral, and after a few weeks I received a letter from CAMHS requesting that the school nurse or the CAMHS representative at the school should assess Mohamed first and then write a report for them, explaining how the school viewed the problem and what help had been given so far.

I was very frustrated by this buck passing and time wasting. I knew that Mohamed needed help now, not in a few months' time. So I decided I had had enough and wrote a stiff letter to both of them to cut out this bureaucracy and to get on with the job. Thankfully it seemed to work and Mohamed was seen and engaged with the service. Initially there were some difficulties because CAMHS assumed that it was all due to bullying and behavioural problems. But eventually they realised how serious his anxiety, depression and detachment disorder were and that he needed a lot of time and hard work to sort out. The emotional scars of the trauma from his past would need help and might need a long time to heal, possibly being carried to his adolescence and later in his life.

Aysha seemed to have suffered fewer traumas and was closer to her mother, joining her on shopping trips, cooking with her in the kitchen, and sometimes going with her to help with the charitable work.

She was relatively happy in school, eager to learn and showing promise in her studies. The only thing that caused her occasional pain was deliberately forgetting her PE kit. Fatima would prepare it for her, leaving it at the front door so she wouldn't forget. But her kit was always in a supermarket plastic bag, while her classmates were all carrying their kits in expensive bags with well-known brand names. She just felt embarrassed but knew that her mum could not afford to buy these things. Sometimes it was just easier to seem forgetful, or have a stomach ache.

* * * * *

Over time I did not see Fatima as often. But one day she came to one of my administration sessions, bringing with her several forms which she needed help with to allow her to claim the support she needed. Despite the fact that I could have asked Sharon or any other administration staff to help her, I preferred to do myself so I could hear about the progress of her and the family.

Fatima told me proudly that Mohamed had grown up into a handsome young man. But then a sad look clouded her face as she mentioned that he had changed a bit too. He now spent a lot more time with his friends, gathering near a coffee shop belonging to a Somali man. It was next to the Halal chicken shop, also owned by same man. Mohamed would eat chicken and chips with his friends and then wouldn't eat at home afterwards.

When Fatima pointed out to him that he didn't eat at home with her and Aysha and spent a lot time with these mates (who she learned later were like a local gang), he answered her that the school always told him to 'nitigrate' in the society. I realised that she meant 'integrate', and Mohamed was doing just that.

The only trouble was that Fatima had no control and had no idea what was going on until one day the school asked to see her. They informed her that Mohamed was part of a group of boys who were suspected of being involved in gang activities like fighting, stealing and taking drugs. The leader, a much older boy, would give them money and 'protection' and they all looked up to him and did anything he asked. They could be identified by the coloured headband they all wore and called themselves the 'African Lions'. They said that Mohamed had not been caught doing anything illegal but that she needed to keep a close eye on him.

This was something that had made her feel very uncomfortable and she decided to monitor the situation and to gather more information first. Then one day she confronted Mohamed. He confessed that it was the other boys and not him who were consuming something called 'Khat', green leaves that release stimulants when chewed and was still very popular in the Somali community, despite now being illegal in the UK. Mohamed couldn't see a problem with this as it only made them calm and happy, nobody got hurt. When Fatima insisted that he stopped seeing these boys Mohamed got very angry. She never saw him like that before. Although he later apologised and said he would stay away, he still left the house making the excuse that he was going to see a friend to study.

Mohamed then started to spend even more time in the street with his friends, not caring what his mum thought or said. When he came home Fatima could smell cigarette smoke on his clothing, but Mohamed just said it was from the friends he sat with in the coffee shop because they smoked cigarettes and Shisha (Middle Eastern hubble bubble). Fatima also started to notice that he seemed to have more money despite the pocket money she gave him would only just pay for a small meal. When she asked him about the money she had found in his trouser pocket before washing them, he explained that he helped out at the coffee shop sometimes and the owner would give him a little cash in hand. Later Fatima learned from some neighbours that the coffee shop owner would send the boys to East London to get the Khat for him so he didn't need to leave the shop. He would give them some pocket money for that.

Fatima was very worried about all these changes. Every time she tried to talk with Mohamed he just shouted at her, got very angry and left the house. Aysha was watching helplessly. She was aware of what Mohamed was doing as some of her friends at the school had brothers who were also involved and they would tell her.

One evening Mohamed came home earlier than usual. He was sweating and was looking worried and frightened. He went straight to his room, not even saying hello. When he was called for supper he was very quiet and reluctant to talk to them, only eating a little before going back to his room.

The next day he refused to go to school and when Fatima asked him why, he finally told her that he was scared to go because he had heard that one of the friends he hung out with had had a fight with a member of another gang and had stabbed him. Thankfully the injured guy had been treated in the hospital and was OK, but now he was scared the other gang might come for revenge on his friends.

Fatima was very frightened and upset and came to me for help. I decided to write to CAMHS to see him for anger management, and the trauma over the recent stabbing. They saw him again for few sessions and then wrote to me that he just came across as a shy, reserved person, who knew his goals, but sometimes got easily irritated. So they offered him some anger management sessions and CBT (Cognitive Behavioural Therapy).

Fatima was relieved that Mohamed agreed to this and he worked hard to improve. It took time to help Mohamed but they were rewarded with good results and he was discharged by CAMHS. Fatima was very happy about the progress, but unfortunately, after a while, he went back to his bad ways.

Mohamed continued to have trouble at school as well. Frequent detentions and temporary exclusions, one after another, caused Fatima much sadness and what confused her was that she couldn't understand that nobody could see her son needed help, not just punishment. Eventually, before the school excluded him permanently, Mohamed and Fatima decided to move him to a different school in the same borough. Luckily he was accepted, but after just a few weeks he had a fight with a boy during the lunch break and ended up in the headmaster's office.

Now Mohamed was on the radar again. The school sometimes did random checks on the pupils, looking for drugs like 'legal' highs and on one of these occasions they found a small kitchen knife in Mohamed's bag. Mohamed immediately denied that it was his, but Fatima recognised it immediately as one from the set in her kitchen. That incident, following on from others, led to headmaster deciding to permanently exclude Mohamed from the school.

The poor Fatima had to go through the whole process of writing to the school governors and to the educational panel (with the help of Aysha) to appeal for some leniency due to the circumstances. However, Fatima noticed that Mohamed didn't really care about the outcome anyway.

Mohamed was excluded, despite Fatima appealing the decision, and Mohamed ended up in alternative education, being sent to a charitable organisation with an educational supervisor. Mohamed joined eight other excluded children from the same borough, but from different schools. He found himself alone among strangers. Looking around the classroom on the first day he spotted the only empty seat available was beside a girl called Emma, who was probably a year younger than Mohamed, with wide blue eyes and light brown hair with red hair extensions. At first she was quiet, answering his questions with single worded answers. In fact she seemed uncomfortable whenever anyone started talking to her. She would bite her nails or chew the end of her hair and look anywhere but at the person talking.

Day after day Mohamed came to talk to her and slowly she seemed to find it easier to talk to him. They found that they had quite a bit in common. Both had had a pretty poor school record and been excluded many times, they shared the same opinions about teachers and hated anything to do with school and discipline. Emma decided to call him "Mo" as the name Mohamed was too much of mouthful for her and he was quite happy with that. He was also happy to meet any of her requests, like buying her cigarettes because she looked too young to buy them herself. It wasn't long before they became good friends. Both of them dreamed of total freedom and independence; a great ambition but one they did not realise carried a lot of heavy responsibilities. As teenagers, young and hopeful but with no life experience they did not estimate or understand the challenges that life could bring.

One day Emma invited Mo to come and say hello to her mum. He was nervous and wanted to make a good impression, but she showed little interest in Mo, apart from saying 'Hello' and telling him that if he wanted a cup of tea the mugs were all in the sink. Mo followed Emma into the cramped messy kitchen and Emma pulled the two least dirty mugs from the sink and rinsed them under the tap. As they left later her mother said nothing and just kept drinking her lager and watching her favourite TV program. Mo never saw Emma's mum again. The following week Emma told Mo that she had had a big row with her mother and had left the house, going to live with her auntie in east London.

I didn't see Fatima or Mohamed for quite some time after that. Fatima came in a few times to see one of our nurses or another clinician for minor ailments, but I wasn't at the clinic on those occasions.

* * * * *

So the little family carried on their lives, the children rapidly growing up into young independent minded people. Aysha loved Mohamed dearly. But despite being very close to Mohamed as they grew up together in the UK, Aysha noticed there had been a drift in Mohamed's thoughts and behaviour. Like her mum she worried about him and felt sad about her brother. Every time she talked to him for an explanation he just found excuses and wouldn't answer her.

One day she was surprised to find Mohamed sitting on her bed looking a bit low. She asked him if he was OK. Mohamed shrugged and at first he just mentioned his discontentment with the school system, and Aysha understood very well how bad a time he had had. Then he told her that he thought going to Friday prayers (something his mum had insisted on since he was old enough to go on his own) was exactly like ticking boxes. The imam had a few topics to talk about that seemed to bear no relevance to the 'real' world. How dare any one of them talk about what was going on in their community, like the drugs and the stabbings or even the horrible events around the world where people were killing and being killed in the name of religions or otherwise. He laughed sarcastically, saying that probably the government was sending an agent to record what the Imam was saying in the Friday prayers, hoping to catch one or two by labelling them as extremists inciting hatred.

Mohamed paused for a while as if he was struggling with a big decision. He took a deep breath and told Aysha he needed to tell her something before telling their mum. Aysha sat on the bed next to him waiting for him to speak. He looked a bit awkward and finally said that he wanted to invite a friend called Emma to say hello, to meet her and their mum. Aysha nodded and said she would let their mum know. Mohamed seemed relieved and kissed her on the forehead before leaving the room. He hadn't done that since they were little.

As promised, Aysha spoke to Fatima later that evening. Both agreed it would be good to meet one of his friends, and it was a positive thing that Mohamed felt able to do so. He had never brought any of his friends home before. Fatima had been afraid that he had might have been ashamed of their humble home. She was happy that things seemed to be changing with Mohamed.

What neither Mohamed nor Fatima knew was that Aysha had already learnt a lot about Emma from the sister of one of Mohamed's friends at the coffee shop. She knew Emma had been excluded from school and left home to live with an aunt in east London. She would meet Mohammed there when he would go to get the Khat for the coffee shop owner. Mohamed would give Emma money and would buy her weed.

However, the visit, though brief, seemed to pass with no incident. Aysha said nothing and just kept observing. She did not want to spoil the obvious pleasure Fatima felt at having this guest, but she did not trust Emma, and worried about the influence she was having on her brother.

A few days later Mohamed had an altercation with his mother because she had noticed he was no longer praying regularly or going to the mosque. Aysha was watching apprehensively, guessing what might come next. When inevitably the subject of traditions and culture came up he bluntly told Fatima to keep her traditions to herself, adding he was sick of being told what to do and think like some child. He said he was going to live with his girlfriend, she didn't like any of those traditions and he didn't feel comfortable with them either.

Fatima had fallen completely silent looking at her son in shock, as if she was seeing a complete stranger. Aysha was furious about how Mohamed had spoken to their mother, but she kept her calm and asked if this was the reason Emma hadn't come back to visit them again. He nodded. But Aysha wasn't finished and asked what exactly it was that Emma didn't like about their traditions.

Mohamed scowled at his sister and started reeling off all the things he could think of. First of all when Emma entered the house they had asked her politely to take her shoes off as no shoes allowed in the house. This had embarrassed Emma as her socks were sweaty and possibly smelly. Emma had tried to be friendly, but struggled with the unfamiliar names. She thought to shorten them, but couldn't really call Mo's mum 'Fat' instead of Fatima, and gave up, just feeling awkward. Then when they had tea they didn't have tea bags like a normal family, just loose tea and a strainer, which how they always had it. They didn't have proper sofas and chairs like other people– just low couches near the floor. He was embarrassed that there was Somali music on the radio, which Emma couldn't understand and was too loud so he had to switch it off. When Emma used the loo, there were no loo paper and she had to use a tissue paper from her pocket. She was shocked to hear that they used a mini shower beside the loo to clean instead of loo paper. Emma also couldn't understand why Fatima and Aysha were wearing head-scarves, even in the house. It was also old-fashioned and primitive in a modern country.

Aysha glared at him as he insulted their hospitality and humble home. But all that she said was that they been brought up to respect other people's cultures and traditions and their freedom to choose what they liked and any civilised person would do the same. She pointed out that their mum and their faith had taught them not to be judgemental or unfair. Maybe Mohamed should think about it.

Mohamed turned his back and went to his room, slamming the door behind him. Aysha hugged her mum, whispering that he didn't mean it, he was just confused. She gently led Fatima to their room and helped her to bed. Then she went back to sitting room and decided to do some research on the internet about some of the points Mohamed had called 'primitive traditions'.

What she discovered was very interesting. These 'traditions' were not just a Somali or Muslim habit. The habit of removing shoes on entering a house was a common practice in many countries, for example, in Japan, which is known for its cleanliness. Japan could never be considered 'primitive', in fact being very technologically advanced. Science and common sense knows that outdoor shoes carry very high levels of bacteria and dirt on the soles, which can be brought into the house and cause contamination.

Aysha was encouraged and moved on to toilet hygiene. She read that medicine had for a long time recommended that it was much healthier to use water rather than tissue to clean the private parts. This because wiping spreads the germs while water carries them away. Incidentally this was also a habit in Japan.

Finally, looking at the headscarf she found this was a practice of modesty that had been and still was in some cases part of both Christian, Jewish, Hindu, Sikh and other faiths and cultures. Researching tea bags, she was surprised to discover that sometimes the chemical epichlorohydrin was used in the manufacture of the bags. This can be harmful to our bodies and the immune system. So if possible it was safer and healthier to use loose tea.

Aysha put all these facts together on one sheet of paper and handed it to her brother, telling him he should at least get his facts right before criticising. Maybe he could educate Emma too. Mohamed read what she gave him, shrugged dismissively and gave it back to Aysha. She looked sadly at her brother, asking him, "Is love blind? Or does it make people blind?"

Mohamed turned away from his sister, knowing she was right. But this just made him angry so grabbed his jacket and escaped the situation by saying that he had to go and see his friends. From that moment on Mohamed used to think twice before saying anything to Aysha and they just drifted further apart.

Fatima and Aysha felt a terrible sadness filling the flat that had once been a happy home. Both of them knew that Mohamed was going on the wrong path and felt helpless watching it happen. Despite Aysha asking her not to say any more, Fatima was desperate to try and change Mohamed's mind.

When Aysha was out at a friend's house, Fatima approached Mohamed and said she understood his frustrations and difficult things he had had to deal with in his young life. She was sorry things had been so hard for them and had done her best to keep them safe. She was just so afraid for him and the people he was mixing with. She knew he was a good person but it wasn't safe to hang around gangs and drugs. Now was not the time to give up on Allah. His father wouldn't have wanted that for him. He would have advised him pay attention to his prayers and spend time with the good people.

Mohamed stared at her as if she had slapped him. Fatima hadn't mentioned his father to him for many years (she had been too afraid to raise the terrible memories of his loss). Now it cut him deeply and he completely lost his temper.

Mohamed started shouting at his mum, saying she had no idea about his life or his friends who really cared about him. Nobody else really cared. Not the school, the teachers, the psychiatrists, the Imams, or anyone. All they cared about was their reputations, inspections and results. The teachers went off sick and were replaced by supply teachers who knew nothing and cared even less. The psychiatrists just ticked boxes and sent you away and the Imams just said what they were told to. Then he accused Fatima and Aysha of caring more about 'tradition' than about him. If it was that important then why had they left Somalia at all? Fatima gasped, but Mohamed was so angry he couldn't stop. He punched the wall and stormed out of the flat, shouting back that he wasn't a child any more and could make his own decisions and didn't need their interference.

I heard about this from Fatima when she came to me for a character reference for her, as she was helping a charity collecting used clothes and donations from around the area. As I did this for her she told me about Mohamed's behaviour and his uncontrolled anger. I was very worried for the young man and asked her to convince him to come and see me. I was relieved when I found his name on my Friday afternoon list.

Mohamed came and I just listened to what happened and his points of view. I accepted that he felt frustrated and let down by the system, but asked him to give me one more chance to find him the right support. He looked so tired and vulnerable despite his anger. He eventually agreed that I would communicate with CAMHS to try to get him an appointment to see them urgently.

It was already approaching 4pm and I wanted to get the ball rolling as quickly as possible and not leave it until Monday morning. But I had a full list of patients to see. So I asked Veronica, our senior admin, to help me out. I briefed her about Mohamed and left the mission with her. I knew she was a fast worker but I was surprised when she popped in between two patients to let me know the outcome.

Veronica had tried to call secretary's office at the Mental Health Trust. She tried several numbers that had been provided by the trust in a recent email announcing their move to shiny new offices. Only one number answered and it was a terrible line. It was answered by an impatient man who had never heard of the secretary. When Veronica asked if there was another number where she could contact the mental health team as this was an urgent matter he just laughed and said how the hell should he know, this was an Indian restaurant and not a telephone directory, and hung up.

Veronica checked she had dialled the number on the email – and yes it was exactly as written. She was very cross, but wondered how many other people had called that guy asking for the mental health team – no wonder he was so grumpy.

But this didn't solve her problem. Veronica called reception to see if they had any other numbers. Janet answered and said yes – there had been a message last week that the new offices had flooded and they were temporarily working at their old offices – so they had their old numbers again.

Veronica finally got in touch with one of the managers, who explained that Mohamed had been discharged from the child mental health service because he was already well over 17 years old, which was the age limit for child services. By the time the referral came through and he had been added to the waiting list, his appointment might not be for a several months. By that time he might have turned 18 and would need to be referred to Adult Mental Health anyway. So he would probably be better off waiting until he turned 18 as adult services were under less pressure and more likely to see him.

When I heard that I held my tongue, so as not to use any inappropriate language. But I was not going to give up on the young man. I had one last trick up my sleeve.

I reminded Veronica about Dr Ferguson, a consultant child psychiatrist from the local Mental Health Trust, who had come to the surgery about two months earlier with his team to speak at our clinical meeting. He had told us that they were collecting feedback about the service in order to try to improve it. When he invited me to comment I asked my clinicians to tell him about the multiple troubles they had had with the service. He was little taken aback by their frankness and when he asked me again I asked him what the point was. Each time we gave feedback and highlighted the gaps in the service, each representative would write it down and nothing would happen. He seemed embarrassed and I felt a bit bad shooting the messenger. But I was surprised when he wrote down his mobile number and said if I ever had a problem I should call him directly and he would sort it out personally for me.

I told Veronica to get me his mobile number from the practice directory and rang Dr Ferguson. I explained the situation to him and he asked me to pass the information to his secretary. I declined politely, asking if at 4:30pm on a Friday she was likely to be there. A pause, and he agreed to write down all the details and promised he would sort it out personally and ensure Mohamed would be seen early next week.

I followed Mohamed's progress through the letters from CAMHS and saw he had a few sessions with them and was then discharged again. I learned that he had applied to a college to do a plumbing course but did not attend regularly. He was still hanging around with his old mates and still seeing Emma. It wasn't the good news I'd hoped for and I felt so sad for Fatima.

* * * * *

One day Fatima came for her medication review and to discuss her fibromyalgia. She looked tired but said she was coping with life's challenges. She smiled and just said 'Alhamdulillah' (thank God) – it was her answer to everything.

Mohamed had ended up in trouble again and Fatima had been called to the local police station, who told her that Mohamed and his mates had been involved in a fight in the coffee shop. Two strangers come to buy some Khat from the owner and disagreed about the price. A scuffle started and soon escalated into a fight. Mohamed tried to protect the owner and hit one of strangers with a massive wooden spoon that had been decorating the wall of the coffee shop. Thankfully it resulted in nothing more serious than a small laceration and was dealt with by the ambulance crew. Fatima hurried to the police station with Aysha, where the first thing she did was go to the injured man to apologize to him. As he raised his head to look at her they both froze. Despite the many years that had passed they immediately recognised each other. It was Ahmed, the young man who had helped Fatima and the children escape from the Calais camp.

They both started speaking at the same time, both shocked and delighted to see each other. In all the mixed emotions she almost forgot herself and was about to hug him, but restrained herself due to her modesty. She almost forgot to introduce Aysha, who was standing by, surprised by what she was seeing and couldn't comprehend what was going on. Fatima explained to Aysha, who could barely remember the time in the camp, and introduced her to Ahmed. Then she remembered that she had come to collect her son.

Ahmed reassured her he wasn't pressing charges and that Mohamed had only been trying to protect his boss. The boss had decided not to say anything as he knew that it was best to avoid any investigation into his activities. He claimed it was a misunderstanding.

Fatima made sure Mohamed apologised and asked forgiveness from Ahmed, a man who had probably saved their lives in helping them come to England.

Fatima invited Ahmed to come for a meal and a chat as he was a very dear and special friend had done so much for Fatima and the family. Ahmed happily accepted the invitation and it was a very nice evening, talking about their past adventures. It was the first time Mohamed and Aysha had heard the full story. They had both been so young at the time and only realised now all the things their mother had been through to bring them to safety in the UK.

Ahmed was very happy to see them all again and agreed that he would be in touch every time he came to London. He was now studying in Manchester to become a surveyor, which was a huge achievement as when he finally arrived in the UK he was very far behind with his education.

* * * * *

I saw Aysha a few months later. She was now starting her last year in school and had applied to study radiography at the local university. She had brought a form for me to sign for her. Fatima had come too and I remember her comment that Aysha loved photography at school and that was why she had chosen radiography.

As promised, Ahmed still came every now and then to visit the family and one day Fatima told me that Ahmed had proposed to Aysha and she had accepted. However, Fatima had insisted Aysha finish her degree before they married, so Ahmed continued to make his regular trips from Manchester.

However, I also noticed that Fatima didn't mention Mohamed a lot any more. When she came on one of her routine visits I asked about Mohamed. Fatima was not at all happy about his progress. He had moved out of the flat and gone to stay in a house with some of his friends. But it was clear that he spent more and more time with Emma in east London. He had deregistered from our clinic, so had found another GP. We got a call one morning asking for a copy of his notes to be sent to a GP in east London, so I guessed he must have finally moved in with Emma and her auntie.

Fatima heard later from friends that Emma had fallen pregnant and the social services were keeping an eye on her due to her vulnerable situation of being a young mother, drinking, smoking and using drugs.

This made Fatima very sad and worse still, Mohamed not even contacted her to tell her the news. In fact he rarely got in touch at all, except maybe to ask for money or when he passed by to see the coffee shop owner to drop some Khat.

When the child was born Fatima learned that the baby girl had been taken into care of Emma's auntie, as Emma had developed severe postnatal depression and was not able to look after her. Things went from bad to worse when Fatima learned that Mohamed had been caught by the police for a drugs-related offence and might have to serve a jail sentence.

Fatima and Aysha then lost touch with Mohamed and assumed he had indeed gone to prison. About a year later they were surprised by a knock at the door during the Eid celebration. It was Mohamed, bearing a small gift for them. Despite his youth he looked like an old man. But to Fatima he was the best Eid present ever. He didn't stay long, but promised he'd come to Aysha's wedding, which he did. But that was the last time either of them ever heard from him again.

* * * * *

Some years later, Fatima came to ask me to fill in the form to apply for a passport as she was planning to visit

Somaliland. While I was filling the forms I found Fatima was in a chatty mood, she was going on and on about 'cycling' and with my concentration focused on the form, my brain only picked up the repeated word of 'cycling'. I thought for a while that she was maybe planning to go cycling to Africa, something I'm sure Fatima would be capable of if she put her mind to it. But when I paid proper attention to what she was talking about, it was the idea of 'recycling' old clothes. She said that she would like to take that idea to Somaliland.

Anyone dealing with Fatima could see that with both her children having left and busy with their own lives, she had started to feel increasingly homesick. She mentioned a long time ago that her older sister had settled in Somaliland because it was much safer than Mogadishu. She had developed severe knee arthritis, which made her mobility difficult, so she couldn't come to London to visit Fatima. So Fatima had decided to visit her instead. She asked me a favour to write down for her the names of some good creams for arthritis that she can buy over the counter and take to her sister and I was glad to help.

Fatima collected her prescription for two months and left for Somaliland. When she returned she had picked up a dry cough from the long flight and the change of environment. She brought me a box of dates which I kindly requested her to give it to the hard-working staff in the reception. She told me about the great time she had had with her sister, but also the sad news about the death of her brother in-law having left her sister feeling very lonely. Fatima hinted that she might think to pack everything up in London and go back to live near her sister. She felt that she has done everything she could for the children, who were both now grown up and living their lives.

She was very happy about Aysha, who had just told her that she had fallen pregnant.

She was, however, less happy about Mohamed. His time in prison had not changed his attitude and he was still doing everything the same. Fatima was about to cry when she said she had not seen him since Aysha's wedding and he rarely called.

She felt she had done everything she could but he was now grown up and didn't take advice from anybody. She said that he reminded her of the story of the Prophet Noah and his son. No matter often Noah advised his son and tried to help him, the boy didn't listen and eventually he lost his life. I felt that indirectly she worried that this might be Mohamed's fate too.

I felt sorry for her and sympathised and consoled her that she had done her very best and that she had extremely well in very difficult circumstances. I think maybe she accepted that and felt reassured.

After a brief pause I looked up again from the form and noticed her face now had a broad smile. She told me that she had a confession to make. Intrigued, I gave her my undivided attention.

She looked for a moment as if the years had fallen from her and she was a shy schoolgirl. She asked me if I remembered the day she had told me that she didn't want to marry again. I nodded. Then she revealed that she had another reason for going back to Somaliland.

While she was there she had been introduced to one of their distant relatives, a man called Ismael. She remembered that when she was a small child he had come with his parents to visit them and they had played together while the adults talked. He was older than her by about three years or so and had married one of his neighbours. He had worked hard as a businessman, had been very successful and became quite wealthy and earned high respect from his tribe for all the good work he had done for them.

Sadly when they had been travelling to Somaliland his poor wife had fallen ill with a fever and weakness. The illness

114

progressed so quickly that she couldn't be saved. As they didn't have any children Ismael decided to start an orphanage and dedicate himself to helping others.

Fatima found that she has lots in common with Ismael and soon they agreed to keep in touch. Before she left to return to London they got engaged in a low-profile ceremony at her sister's house.

Fatima said she had told the children as soon as she got back and both Mohamed and Aysha were very happy for her. I added my congratulations on her wonderful news. She smiled and said that sometimes we think we can make a decision in life, like saying we will never marry, but sometimes God has different ideas...and they are always right!

Later on I learned from Aysha that Fatima had opened a charity shop in Somaliland with the help of Ismael to sell second-hand clothes sent from London and Manchester with the help of Ahmed and many of their friends. They money raised was given to the orphanage to provide an education for the children.

* * * * *

One day I was attending an educational meeting at our local hospital, where Aysha now worked as a radiographer. Aysha saw me and came over to tell me all the news about her mum, who was very happily married and settled in Somaliland. Her charity shop had done really well and they had now opened two more in different parts of the country, along with another orphanage. Fatima Abdullah had also become quite an important person in Somaliland. She was well respected for giving excellent advice to people due to her vast experience in Europe and in life in general. She also learned to drive and bought a small car, spent some time teaching English to the orphans and helping the poor and needy refugees coming from Somalia.

Aysha also mentioned that she was leaving the local hospital and had applied for a job in Manchester so she and Ahmed could be to be closer to his uncle, who was getting older and needed care.

Later on I realised that all the family had now been deregistered from our list. I was sad to see them all go, but I always remember them with a smile.

Fatima left me with a strong feeling of respect and humbleness to this remarkable woman, who faced many challenges and overcome them, she was supported by her very strong faith and determination, it was a great privilege to know her and her little family.

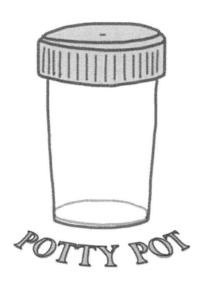

POTTY POT

Chapter 6

In our surgery in South-East London, and in general, life used to be simpler over the past two decades, with no security alerts and requests to change the password for the work computer every month or so, making sure to choose a complex selection of letters, numbers, symbols etc. Not only that, but we are instructed to remember this combination every time we log in, as the computer is not allowed to save it for us for security reasons.

Adding to these challenges of working life, we sometimes get new instructions from the decision makers (some managers like to change things every now and then) just for the sake of it. It doesn't matter whether they make sense or not.

We used to have many electronic forms on our computer system, accompanied by a master copy in the main office. These forms are usually one or two pages long and we use them to make referrals to different services. However, it has come to our attention in the last decade or two that these services have a habit of repeatedly changing the forms, every time becoming longer, more complex, and more daunting to fill in for doctors and administration staff (it's as though somebody thought the level of bureaucracy should be increased in line with inflation!)

Then suddenly – whoops! – There's not much time left for the care of our patients.

But I'll stop moaning about the forms now as it seems the computer has crashed again. Looking on the bright side, it's probably just being kind to us, to give us a break.

* * * * *

One day while I was thinking about these computer issues, the outdated system we are using, and the repeated empty promises from the Trust, that they are going to update the system, Veronica (our senior administrator) came to tell me she'd received a call from the pathology laboratory of the University Hospital in central London asking her two questions; why our staff were not giving patients coming from our surgery the pot they needed to use to provide a sample for semen analysis; and why we weren't using the new forms?

Thankfully I realised what she was talking about, as I had seen a young Nepalese patient in his early thirties two days earlier, and I requested the test. My patient, Mr Gurung, whom I had known for years, was a shy and polite patient. He had a business degree and was working for a reputable company in the city. He had married in a fabulous ceremony and his mother had showed me the videos on her mobile phone.

Mr Gurung and his wife came to see me, as they had been trying for a baby for more than two years, without success. Due to pressure from the family, he had come to ask for some investigations to be done for him and his wife.

He needed to give a semen sample for analysis; so I printed the form from the computer, completed it and went through it with him – there was a page with instructions for him to follow and a number for him to ring the main laboratory at the University Hospital in London to make an appointment. The other part of the form was for the surgery to fax to the main lab to request the test, and I referred his wife to the fertility clinic.

In the past, this specific test of semen analysis used to be done in our local hospital, which was very convenient for our patients. We used to give the patient the pot, which had been supplied by the local hospital, so they could provide a sample in the comfort of their own home, and then they would take it to the hospital in less than half-an-hour to be processed (samples MUST be brought to the hospital within one hour of production).

However, now the contract had been changed, so that this specific test had to be done at the main laboratory of the University Hospital in London. This lab was much further away than the one in the local hospital and it would certainly take more than an hour to get there, which could affect the sample and is far less convenient for the patient.

So Mr Gurung had gone to have his test in the morning and Veronica had received the call from a lady called Mrs Wilde, working at the central laboratory of the University Hospital.

Veronica had a puzzled gaze and a little frown on her face, as if she had been tearing her hair out, and said: "I told Mrs Wilde that we had stopped giving pots to the patients about a year ago, since the contract had been changed for this service. The advice given at that time was that it was not appropriate for the patient to give the sample at home then take it all the way to the central lab, a journey which would take more than an hour by any means of transport. Over that time the sample would be affected and the results would be inaccurate. So the practical way was for the patient to report to the central laboratory, and be given a pot by them to do a fresh and viable sample there."

Mrs Wilde had replied that they had changed management recently and the new protocol was for the GP surgery to get the pots from the central lab at the university and to give it to the patient, who would take it back to the central lab to provide a sample there.

She added that our form was out of date and she would send us the new one, together with another form for ordering the pots from the central lab.

Veronica asked Mrs Wilde to fax us the new form, so we could scan it and keep it on our computer for future use. Mrs Wilde said very firmly that she would email it, as they don't fax nowadays because the government target is to move towards a paperless policy.

Veronica patiently tried to explain that the email service was down and that our computers had crashed. The IT engineers were working on it but we don't know when it was going to be functioning again.

So Veronica rang the central laboratory and told them about the issue. To her surprise, they said that they were not able to supply these pots directly to GPs, as they only sent them to local hospitals, so we would need to order them from there!

I looked at Veronica and realised that we still hadn't sorted the problem. Meanwhile, Mr Gurung had also called the surgery from the University Hospital to report the problem of the pot. He had a relative working as a nurse in the same hospital, so he called him for help. This relative had no luck with the pathology reception staff, adding more frustration to poor Mr Gurung, who had dedicated that whole day to the test, as he had used up all his holidays. He'd taken unpaid leave and couldn't afford to take another day off, with his wife not working, so he asked our staff for help.

By that time I realised that this pot problem was driving everybody potty, and decided to do something about it myself.

I rang the central lab at the University Hospital and asked to talk to the manager, only to be told he was in a meeting and I would have to leave a message. I had no time for this, as by now I had a session to run, and the patients were waiting. I asked to speak to his deputy, Mr Logan.

I introduced myself and explained the issue of the pots. He understood the complexity of the problem and agreed to raise it with the senior managers at the next meeting. I only just kept my temper, and explained again that Mr Gurung was at the University Hospital right now and couldn't wait until the next meeting!

Thankfully, Mr Logan agreed to personally arrange for a pot to be provided to Mr Gurung and for our surgery to be exempted from supplying the pots. He also agreed that we could continue to use the old forms for now.

I was pleased with that outcome and a few days later I reviewed the results of Mr Gurung, which were satisfactory, and the subject faded away from my memory.

Some months later, Alisha, our nurse, called me for a routine eight weeks check for baby Gurung. When I entered the nurse's room and greeted the parents, I remembered Mr and Mrs Gurung and their infertility problem of the past. I congratulated them and I was happy that they had got what they wanted.

I completed the examination and everybody was happy with the outcome. I left the room with a smile. Walking down the corridor back to my room, I remembering vividly the Potty Pot saga, and kept smiling, as we were triumphant in the potty pot battle, against one of many bureaucratic hoops we have to jump through.

That is, of course, until there another change in management, and the merry-go-round of life in the NHS will carry on.

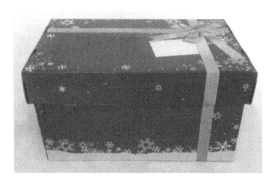

Chapter 7
Unexpected guest

It was an extraordinarily busy Friday at the clinic, being the weekend before Christmas. Some patients were going away and needed last-minute prescriptions, while others were booking an emergency appointment for something they'd had all-year round, like itchy toes from eczema or athlete's foot, which they'd already been given treatment and instructions for – but never followed. Of course we wouldn't ask, 'Why now?'

Some patients started having symptoms of poor sleep caused by the stress of the festive season or unpleasant memories of 'Christmas past'. Demand for sleeping tablet prescriptions reached a record high and would be high-lighted to us by the Trust's team of medicine management in the New Year – good news for shareholders of the pharmaceutical companies.

At last I was pleased to finish the long day and drove home. There I found my hard-working wife, having finished the last-minute shopping, finalising the list of cards which had not been sent yet, and those in response to unexpected cards from people we'd briefly met during trips abroad and promised to stay in touch with.

Then there was the wrapping of additional presents for people who had not been on our gifts list last year, like new in-laws, new boyfriends or girlfriends joining the extended family, and new neighbours.

By now I was getting tired of it all and had lost my enthusiasm, but I was very proud of my wife carrying on with the frantic activity.

The weekend started on a reasonably happy note, with everyone having their own 'to do' list. While we were having breakfast, my wife mentioned with a smile that she needed to rush to the post office and then to the hairdressers to have her hair done for the festive season, to have a new look for the new year – and for me as well.

I was left to finish my cup of tea and to read the newspaper in peace. But not for long as I heard the doorbell ring. I thought it might be another delivery for my wife, who had taken up a new habit of online shopping. So I was surprised to find Alisha, our practice nurse at the surgery, on the doorstep.

I welcomed her with a puzzled smile, as she had never visited us before and, as far as I knew, she did not know our address. Then I realised I'd given it to her a few months earlier, when she'd been under a lot of stress at work, offering to invite her and her husband for a cup of tea and chat to see how we could help. In the end she declined and I supported her as best as I could, and she was happy with a brief chat at work instead.

So here she was, on our doorstep, carrying a huge box and wearing a huge smile.

"Come in, Alisha," I said. But she shook her head and said she was rushing back to her husband, who was waiting in the car. She promised to come another time, but needed to hurry as they had many people and relatives to visit. She pushed the heavy parcel inside the porch and ran down the front garden path, leaving me quite speechless and trying to take in what had happened.

Little did I know that the surprises were not over yet. It started with Buzz the cat coming to see what all the excitement was about and what that new smell in her territory was. Rubbing against my leg, she gave me an inquisitive look, as if to say, 'What's inside the box?'

Being very curious myself, I decided to open the parcel – and thank God I did! If I had just put it under a Christmas tree, with the rest of presents to be opened on Christmas Day, then it would have been a disaster. Because inside the box was a huge frozen turkey, with all its accompanying vegetables, gravy, stuffing, mince pies, Christmas pudding and chocolates. In fact an entire family Christmas dinner in a box!

Still in shock, I was puzzled as to what I should do with this (rapidly defrosting) beast, especially as my wife had already been busy preparing a Christmas beast of our own. I decided it would be best to wait for my wife to come home and consult her about this surprise. Thankfully she returned after a short while.

My wife was equally shocked at this news and exclaimed that the big freezer was already full, as was the fridge; there wasn't even space for a little sparrow, let alone a huge turkey.

Racking her brain, my smart wife came up with an idea – food banks! In a race against time to find a new home for our unexpected guest, everyone got on their phones and we called the nearest, and then the furthest, food banks. But all our enquiries were met with disappointing results. Either the number was not recognised or the food bank had no contact number, only an address. Some of them answered but didn't have a freezer or a fridge to store a turkey, accepting only dry or canned food.

Next we tried a list of our relatives and friends, but this had been exhausted by midday. By now we were behind in our daily schedule, so my wife decided to try to reshuffle the fridge, taking all the food out, removing the upper shelf and rearranging everything inside. But with the turkey squeezed in, you couldn't even see the light at the back of the fridge any more.

We decided it wasn't the end of the world, as we now had a bit more time to deal with this unexpected guest. With no takers so far, we finished for the evening and decided to go to bed and sleep on the problem – hoping for inspiration in the morning.

However, in the middle of the night my wife woke up suddenly and shouted, 'The turkey!'

I thought she was dreaming (or having a nightmare), but she hurriedly explained that she had put the turkey on the top shelf of the fridge and it would by now be gradually defrosting. I frowned and asked her what the problem was.

She stared at me in exasperation, saying, "It will dribble on to the food below! I will have to move it on to the lowest shelf, but that means I will have to reshuffle the whole fridge again."

I looked at her suspiciously and my sleepy brain picked up the word 'reshuffle', as in 'government reshuffle'. I was about to say, 'No, please, no need for a reshuffle, it's the middle of the night'. But soon I realised that my wife was sensible, and would do the reshuffle of the turkey appropriately, putting it in its right place instead of the upper shelf. So she went off the kitchen and, half-asleep, sorted the turkey out. While doing so, she woke up the kids unintentionally, and shouted at them to go back to sleep. The yelling woke me up again at the same time.

Preoccupied with her urgent mission, and eager to get back to bed, she then forgot to close the kitchen door. Seeing the mistake, Buzz the cat thought it was morning and decided to escape from the kitchen. She crept into my room and with her distinctive morning "meow" broke the silence of the night and interrupted my sleep (yet again!)

In frustration at this constant interruption to my sleep, I found myself cursing the b***** turkey for all the chaos.

Thankfully it was Sunday, and the whole family, including Buzz, were able to compensate with a bit of a lie-in. But my wife had other ideas, taking the turkey dilemma as a personal challenge.

She looked very puzzled and said, "I can't believe it. Normally, when you are offering people something extra for free they will immediately say 'yes please'. But with this turkey, everybody is declining it, one after another, as if we were offering them a ticking bomb!"

The search for someone in need of a turkey continued throughout the morning, extending to the kids asking their friends too, as it was becoming a desperate situation (serious defrosting had by now set in).

We then started looking for a recipient among our neighbours, trying to work out who had gone abroad for the holidays , who didn't have their cars in the drive, who was Indian or Sikh (no point in asking them). Another Muslim neighbour probably wouldn't take it unless it was halal!

Eventually my wife had a eureka moment, saying, "I know! Catherine, five doors down the road, might take it, as they are a big family." She searched for a Christmas card and a box of chocolates left in the cupboard and made her way to Catherine's house. Thankfully they were there, my wife was invited in and she told Catherine about the unexpected Christmas guest, and asked if she'd care to have an extra turkey.

Catherine answered, "We'd love to – but we are all vegetarians!"

Seeing the disappointed look on my wife's face, Catherine's partner John stepped in and said, "I can't promise, but I know my Mum may cook it for charity." He phoned his mother and she agreed to take the big beast.

My wife returned to our house like a rocket, in case the deal fell through, and with a triumphant smile she said, "The turkey is going! Cheers!"

She raced to the kitchen, put the turkey back in his big box – and we waved it goodbye.

We decided to thank Alisha very much for her gift and to tell her about our New Year's Resolution – our whole house had decided to go VEGETERIAN.

We agreed never to tell Alisha what had really happened to the turkey (you could call it our fowl play!), until perhaps one day she might read this chapter in this book after I presented a copy to her, with a very wide smile.

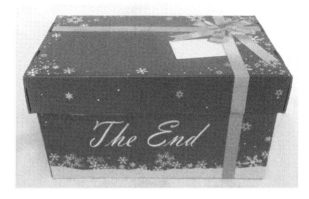

The prequels

If you enjoyed this book, you may like to read the first two in the 'Drops Of Reality' series. Both volumes are available in paperback and Kindle from Amazon.

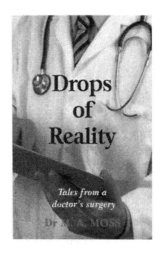

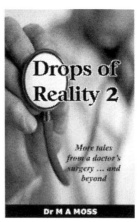

Printed in Poland
by Amazon Fulfillment
Poland Sp. z o.o., Wrocław

61926252R00074